AN ILLUSTRATED GUIDE TO VETERINARY CARE OF THE HORSE

Colin J. Vogel, BVetMed, MRCVS

Gillham House Veterinary Group, Fakenham,

Norfolk, England

Iowa State University Press/Ames

First published in the United States of America in 1996 by Iowa State University Press, 2121 South State Avenue, Ames, Iowa 50014-8300.
ISBN: 0-8138-2080-4

Library of Congress Cataloging-in-Publication Data applied for.

73 Corringham Road, London NW11 7DL, UK.
ISBN: 1-874545-03-0

Colour reproduction by Reed Reprographics, Ipswich, England.
Typeset by Neil Straker Creative, Bishop's Stortford, England.
Printed by Grafos S.A., Barcelona, Spain.

Contents

Dedication

This book is dedicated to Michael Clayton, Editor of Horse and Hound Magazine, who has given me so much encouragement over the years to put my pen to paper.

Acknowledgements

The majority of the colour illustrations in this book were supplied by the Equine Unit of Liverpool University Veterinary School. A donation from the royalties on the sale of the book will be made to the unit, which is a major centre for equine veterinary research.

Additional illustrations were supplied by the Thoroughbred Breeders Association Research Unit *Figs. 99, 101, 102* (pages 93, 96, 97), The Royal Veterinary College *Figs. 111, 112* (page 115), MSD Agvet *Figs. 72, 77, 78, 79, 85, 88, 89, 90* (pages 65, 71, 72, 77, 81, 82), and Boehringer Ingleheim *Figs. 41 & 42* (page 40).

Foreword

Textbooks about the veterinary care of horses have been available for more than a century. In the past, these texts usually were written by veterinarians for lay people who had varying degrees of knowledge about equine health. Historically, such texts were updated only once every 30 or 40 years.

Today, veterinary medical knowledge is vast and rapidly changing, which presents a challenge for both horse owners and veterinarians. Keeping pace with new developments and assessing their value is increasingly demanding.

Also, in today's world medical and veterinary information is widely available in the popular press. Horse owners and trainers are frequently exposed to information regarding health and disease, but often do not have access to information that provides a balanced view of equine health matters in an understandable form, free of medical jargon.

Colin Vogel has compiled a comprehensive and thorough book for the horse owner. It provides valuable information about health care and diseases of horses. Not only will it help horse owners understand their horses' problems, it can help them decide when to seek professional help. It also will help them understand the possible results of many problems. This is not a text that will transform the horseperson into a veterinarian. Rather it will help horse owners and veterinarians work together for the benefit of the horse.

Colin Vogel is to be congratulated for developing a text that acknowledges the knowledge and skills of equine owners and trainers and fosters cooperation between them and their veterinarians. Anyone who works with horses, either professionally or as a hobby, will find this book an invaluable aid and will use it on a day-to-day basis.

Christopher M. Brown, BVSc., PhD, MRCVS,
Diplomate, American College of Veterinary Internal Medicine
Professor, Iowa State University College of Veterinary Medicine

Preface

It has long been my ambition to write a book which would provide the ordinary horse owner with an easy-to-use reference work covering all of the common veterinary problems which can affect the horse. Modern technology has at last made it possible directly to combine colour illustrations and text in a meaningful way. In the text, I have used the nineteenth century term 'veterinarian' rather than veterinary surgeon or vet because it is in more common usage around the world.

Postscript

Veterinary knowledge is increasing at a phenomenal rate. In the equine sphere research is so active that authors have to wait for months or years for there to be a space for their results to be published in major scientific journals such as the Equine Veterinary Journal. As a result there are diagnostic and therapeutic techniques which are evolving as this book goes to press, but which are not included in the main text.

Nuclear Resonance Scanning, for example, is starting to be possible in the anaesthetised horse. This enables us to look at all kinds of tissue and to see the anatomy as a whole, rather than taking X-rays to look at bones, ultrasound scans to look at tendons etc. Who knows where this new ability will take us?

The race is on to devise equipment to enable us to stabilise fractures of the major bones at the top to the horse's leg. This achievement is tantalizingly close, and when the last few problems are solved will have the potential to save many lives.

It is likely that in the future vaccines will become available against a wider range of infections. Work continues on genetically engineered vaccines especially to achieve this. The perfect vaccine against a viral infection does not yet exist, but a lot of basic research is being carried out that will hopefully one day enable us to produce solid, long lasting protection against diseases such as Equine Herpes Virus and Equine Influenza Virus.

I must also strike a pessimistic note. Increasing regulation of the pharmaceutical field has caused the loss of many effective equine products. The result has been that there are often situations where we can cure a horse only if we act 'illegally' and use drugs which we are theoretically not allowed to use for the purpose. There just are not enough horses to make it economic for pharmaceutical companies to spend vast sums on developing and licensing horse products.

Hopefully man's ingenuity will continue to solve the problems posed by equine disease. We owe it to the horses we love to make sure that these advances are applied as widely and as effectively as possible. I hope this book will help in a small way to inform owners about what we can and can't do to help when injury or disease strike.

C. J. Vogel

1: Introduction

A guide to the diseases of the horse must provide help and advice for many different types of horse owner in a variety of situations. So it is appropriate to start with some advice on how best to use this book.

The book is divided into sections rather than chapters. Each section deals with a different system within the horse's body – for example, the digestive system or the reproductive system. At the start of each section is a description of the structure and anatomy of a particular system, and this is followed by a consideration of how the system is adapted to fight disease or injury.

The skin, for example, is obviously a physical barrier to the entry of disease. When that barrier is breached, infection can enter the body. The lining of the stomach also provides a physical barrier against the entry of infection, but, as I will describe later, it also uses chemicals, antibodies and waves of contraction to prevent infections from establishing themselves. You cannot properly understand a specific disease condition unless you already understand the ways in which the horse will try to counteract the condition. This is followed by a brief survey of ways in which you can help to prevent problems and a list, in alphabetical order, of the diseases that affect that part of the body.

You should read the first part of *every* section, to obtain a general introduction on how each part of the horse functions. The details of the individual diseases can then either be browsed through or examined more closely later if you suspect that your horse has a particular problem or if you want more information about a disease that your veterinarian has already diagnosed. Each individual disease is discussed in the same way. First the symptoms are described. Then the cause of the problem is discussed. Thirdly, the various possible treatments are given. Finally the prognosis is made.

'Prognosis' may be an unfamiliar term: it means 'the likely outcome', assuming that the disease is treated promptly with the correct drugs.

A tradition has grown up in medical science that a good prognosis means that the animal will almost certainly recover completely from the ailment and return to normal.

A fair prognosis means that there is a reasonable chance of complete recovery, but some animals may only partly return to normal and a small percentage may not recover at all.

A guarded prognosis means that it is not really possible to say whether the animal will recover or not – in other words, the odds are starting to be stacked against complete recovery. An example of this would be tetanus in a horse whose vaccination programme was not up to date. There is a chance that such a horse might recover, but the majority of horses which get tetanus die.

A poor prognosis means that there is little or no chance of a complete recovery. A horse which has never been vaccinated against tetanus would have a poor prognosis for recovery if it contracted the disease.

The prognosis for a disease can change drastically. Originally the prognosis for any generalised bacterial infection was poor. The discovery, first of penicillin and then of many more antibiotics has changed that, so that for most such cases the prognosis is now good.

Lameness caused by navicular disease was at one time incurable. The discovery of the painkiller phenylbutazone meant that many affected horses could return to work, although they were not cured because they needed continuous medication. The use of new drugs such as isoxsuprine means that the prognosis is now fair, since many horses can return to normal work without needing further medication when the initial course has been completed.

Throughout the book you will find hundreds of symptoms of disease; that is, ways in which there is a change from the normal healthy horse.

The healthy horse

You will only recognise something as being abnormal if you know what a normal healthy horse looks like, how it feels to your touch, and how it functions. Every owner must be familiar with their own horse. Great racehorse trainers owe part of their success to knowing their horses. They react instantly to slight heat and swelling around a tendon or the first couple of coughs in the stable. 'Ordinary' horse owners should be like 'extraordinary' trainers in this respect.

The drugs we use

A general introduction to the most commonly used families of drugs follows. Most of the drugs mentioned in the book are prescription only medicines, available only from your veterinarian or from a pharmacy on prescription. The range of drugs on general sale varies greatly from country to country.

Antibiotics

Antibiotics kill the bacteria that cause infections. There are no drugs licensed for horses which kill viruses. Antibiotics may kill just a narrow range of bacterial species, as in the case of penicillin, or they may be so-called broad spectrum antibiotics that have some activity against a wide range of bacterial families. Oxytetracycline is a broad spectrum antibiotic.

By and large it is better to use a specific antibiotic; culturing and identifying the bacteria in a laboratory, and carrying out sensitivity tests indicate the specific antibiotic to use. So, if we do not know which bacteria is involved we may have to use a broad spectrum antibiotic, but if we have been able to culture and identify the specific bacterium in a laboratory and carry out drug sensitivity tests *(Fig. 1)*, we can target treatment much more precisely.

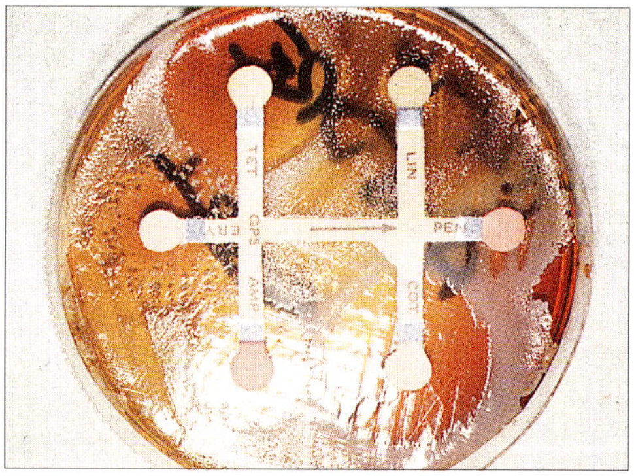

Fig. 1 *Antibiotic Sensitivity Plate*
The six discs are each impregnated with a different antibiotic. Discs surrounded by a clear area have no bacterial growth and so should be effective drugs.

Bacteria may eventually develop resistance to antibiotics, which causes them to lose their efficacy. Giving inadequate doses, or not giving a full course of treatment, can encourage the development by successive generations of bacteria of antibiotic resistance. A wound, for example, may be infected with a strain of bacteria which is already resistant to all the common antibiotics before any treatment has been attempted.

Antibiotics can only work if they actually come into physical contact with the bacteria. Sometimes inflammation and reaction around the site of the infection may prevent adequate quantities of the drug penetrating to where it is needed. By and large, antibiotics do not penetrate well into joints and into the bone marrow, so infections of these parts of the body are particularly serious. Owners sometimes refer to one antibiotic as being 'stronger' than another. This is not a particularly useful method of assessing effectiveness—antibiotics are not relatively stronger or weaker, because in the right circumstances they can all effectively kill bacteria. The veterinarian, faced with a situation where an antibiotic is not working clinically, changes to a different drug rather than a stronger one.

Corticosteroids

Corticosteroids reduce inflammation. They were developed from a substance called cortisone which is used by all mammals to control the body's automatic response to injury of any kind. Because they reduce both good and bad responses, care has to be taken when using corticosteroids in the presence of infection. Corticosteroids reduce the body's ability to fight infection, so they are often accompanied by an antibiotic if there is any suggestion that there might be an associated infection.

Corticosteroids do not, of themselves, remove pain, although it may be reduced as the inflammatory reaction comes under control. In the past they were routinely injected directly into joints to counteract the inflammation associated with arthritis. The improvements can be striking in the short term. Unfortunately, as we now realise, in the long term such injections can predispose to even more serious bone damage, and their use in joints now tends to be a last resort. In ponies particularly corticosteroids can trigger laminitis. They can also cause problems in old horses and pregnant mares.

Non-steroidal anti-inflammatory drugs

Non-steroidal anti-inflammatory drugs (NSAIDs) are among the most widely used drugs in horses. The best known of these is phenylbutazone, otherwise known as 'bute', which was the first member of the group to be discovered, and is by far the cheapest to use. Other NSAIDs include meclofenamic acid, flunixen and naproxen.

These drugs act in two ways. They are analgesics, or painkillers, and they are also anti-inflammatory. When we use such a drug in a horse and see a beneficial response, we do not know whether we have merely removed the pain or whether we have actually speeded up the healing process. Only by withdrawing the drug and seeing whether the pain returns can we discover which action has been the important one. We must be careful when using painkillers. They may encourage the horse to carry out activities which may be detrimental to the underlying condition. Physical wear and tear, such as arthritis, can continue to take place even though the horse appears sound. This brings nearer the day when the condition has progressed so far that no amount of drugs can mask the pain.

Another problem with NSAIDs is that they are to some extent toxic. This is almost always due to their causing ulcers to form on the lining of the intestines. The horse loses vital proteins through these ulcerations, and may even die. Ponies are much more susceptible than horses to such toxicity because their intestinal contents pass along the intestine more slowly.

For years phenylbutazone was thought to be completely safe. It was only after pioneering work by Dr David Snow that the relatively low safety margin for the drug was demonstrated. In the interests of horse welfare in the widest sense, NSAIDs should never be used unless a definite veterinary diagnosis has been made for the horse's condition. The recommended dose should never be exceeded, and if prolonged treatment is needed in small ponies, regular blood tests should be carried out to ensure that the pony is not losing too much protein. It should be appreciated that it takes two or three days for an NSAID administered orally to reach effective levels in the bloodstream.

There is therefore no value in giving a course lasting one or two days, or in dosing less frequently than every other day. Also, the effect of a drug may persist for several days after it has been withdrawn. It is sometimes a good idea to take a blood sample from a horse at purchase so that if necessary tests can be carried out for any NSAID which may have been used to mask lameness.

Vaccines

Vaccines stimulate the horse's natural defence mechanisms in such a way as to enable it to withstand an attack by a particular infection, even though it has never suffered the infection before. Almost always this involves stimulating the horse's body to manufacture large amounts of the specific antibody which can kill the infection. Vaccination needs to be repeated at regular intervals in order to boost the antibody levels. Horse owners seem to expect all vaccines to last for a year before they need repeating. This is unrealistic because the length of time a horse remains immune from infection after even a natural attack of a disease varies greatly. Immunity against equine herpes virus, for example, may only last three to four months after a natural attack, which is why it is proving so difficult to develop a vaccine which will protect the horse for at least a year.

There are two basic kinds of vaccine: live and dead. As its name implies, a live vaccine is manufactured from a living organism which has been altered in some way so that it will stimulate immunity without causing clinical symptoms. A dead vaccine is made from all or part of a disease organism. Usually only one initial dose of a live vaccine is needed, whereas two or three doses of dead vaccines are necessary before they provide adequate protection. Live vaccines tend to be very effective at stimulating immunity but they cause far more side-effects (including clinical disease) than do dead ones *(Fig. 2)*.

Vaccines can protect against both bacteria, such as tetanus, and viruses, such as equine influenza. So far there are no vaccines against worm infections in the horse, but these may become a practical proposition in the future. It is possible to produce combined vaccines against both bacteria and viruses (for example, equine influenza and tetanus). Indeed, in dogs vaccines often provide cover against five different diseases. A recent development has been the manufacture of ISCOM (Immune Stimulating COMplex) vaccines, which contain only the small fragment of the virus that is most effective in stimulating antibody production rather than the whole virus. They appear to be as effective as a whole virus vaccine rather than dramatically better.

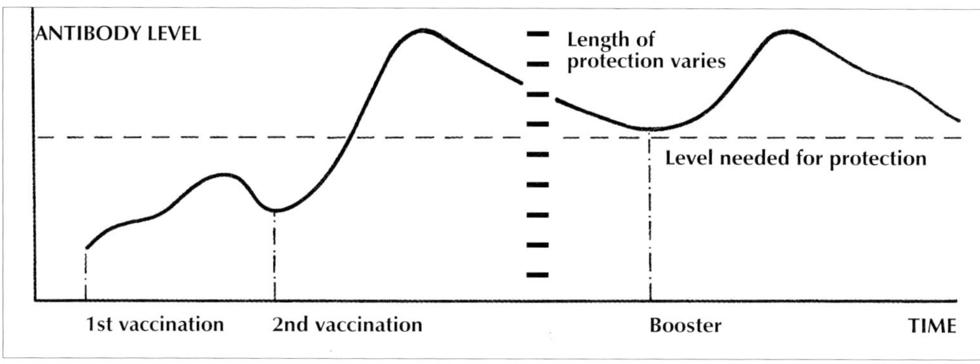

Fig. 2 *The effects of vaccination*

Anaesthesia and sedation

Nerve block

This is a technique used to remove sensation in an area of the body, either to localise the site of pain or to enable some painful procedure to be carried out. Local anaesthetic is injected around the nerve trunk, and absorbed by the nerve. When successfully carried out, sensation in the area normally supplied by the nerve is lost within about 20 minutes of the injection. The length of time for which this lasts varies with the drug used, but is usually only an hour or so. The commonest nerve blocks used are those which remove sensation from the foot and lower leg.

Sedation

There are a number of drugs which make a resting horse sleepy. Only three in common use (romifidine, detomidine and xylazine) can make an already excited horse sleepy and unresponsive. These drugs need to be given by injection. Even so, horses can still kick out with surprising accuracy when stimulated, although this may be controlled by the addition of further drugs. Sedatives have relatively little pain-reducing effect. With the exception of romifidine they also tend to make the sedated horse stagger.

General anaesthesia

For complete relaxation and absence of movement, a general anaesthetic is needed. General anaesthetics have improved tremendously over the past 25 years, and the inherent risk they pose has been reduced accordingly. Anaesthesia is usually produced initially by the intravenous injection of a short acting anaesthetic. This may be all that is required if the operation is a short one. If a longer period of anaesthesia is required a tube may be inserted into the horse's trachea (windpipe), and a mixture of oxygen and a gaseous anaesthetic supplied direct to the lungs. Despite these developments there is always some risk associated with a general anaesthetic. Your veterinarian may ask you to sign a form declaring that you understand the risks involved. You should also notify the insurance company if surgery under general anaesthetic is contemplated on an insured horse.

Diagnostic techniques

Radiography

X-rays have been used for many years. They highlight bony problems, although some softer tissues may be visible, depending on the amount of exposure. X-rays are two-dimensional, and give no indication of depth. Damage to a bone, for example, may be on the side facing the X-ray machine or on the side facing the X-ray plate, but the picture will be the same. A second X-ray taken at an angle of ninety degrees to the first is needed to show which position is actually correct. Most veterinary practices can X-ray a horse's legs as far as the elbow or stifle. Radiography of the chest, abdomen, spine and pelvis requires an extremely powerful X-ray machine usually only found in universities and other institutions *(Fig. 3)*.

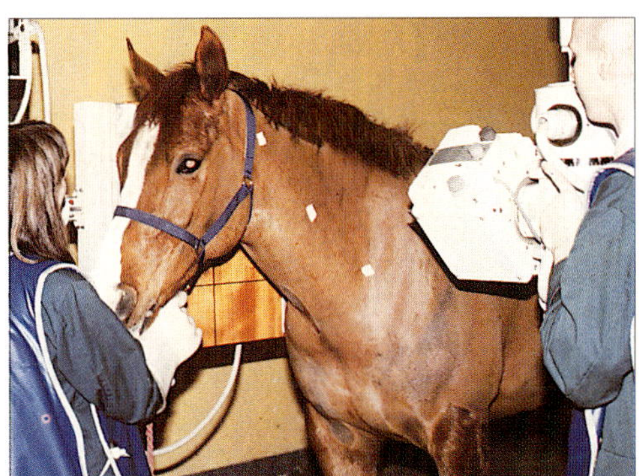

Fig. 3 *X-raying a horse*
A powerful machine which can penetrate even the thickest parts of the horse's body is used.

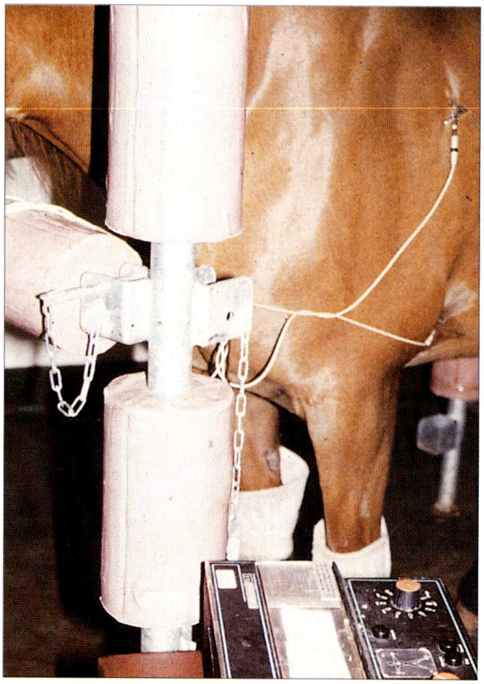

Fig. 4 *Taking an ECG*
Wires lead from the machine to each of the electrodes attached to the horse's skin.

Electrocardiogram

An electrocardiogram (ECG) is a visual reproduction of the electrical activity in the heart. As such it bears no direct relationship to the heart sounds heard with a stethoscope because these reflect blood flow. It is obtained by attaching three or four electrodes to the horse's body and obtaining a reading of the minute electrical forces present *(Fig. 4)*. An ECG provides information about the size and position of the heart, and about its rhythm. The paper record of this information which it provides can be studied and measured for minute abnormalities. The paper trace can even be sent away for specialist evaluation without moving the horse.

Echography

This new technique enables us to see organs at work within the body with much greater clarity than has been possible until now. A scanning probe emits a beam of ultrasound waves, and measures the echoes reflected back from the varying densities of tissue. The resulting composite cross-sectional view of the area can be viewed on a computer monitor. The changes occurring in tendons and other structures can be assessed visually as they heal.

Endoscopy

An endoscope is a long tube, now usually flexible, which is inserted into the horse's body. A bright light is shone down part of the tube while the operator looks at what is being illuminated via fibreoptic strands in another part of the tube *(Fig. 5)*. Using an endoscope passed up a horse's nostril, the airway as far down as the entrance to the lungs can be examined. An arthroscope is a specialised endoscope which is used to look into joints and to carry out microsurgery *(Fig. 6)*.

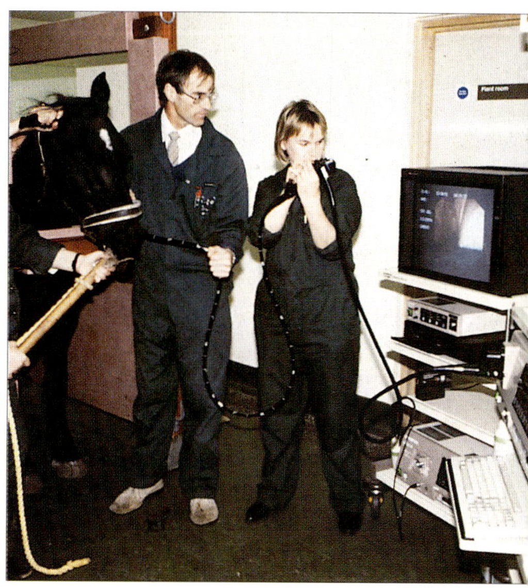

Fig. 5 *Examining a horse's respiratory tract using a video endoscope*
A video camera photographs the image transmitted from inside the horse via optical fibres. The image can be viewed on screen or stored on tape.

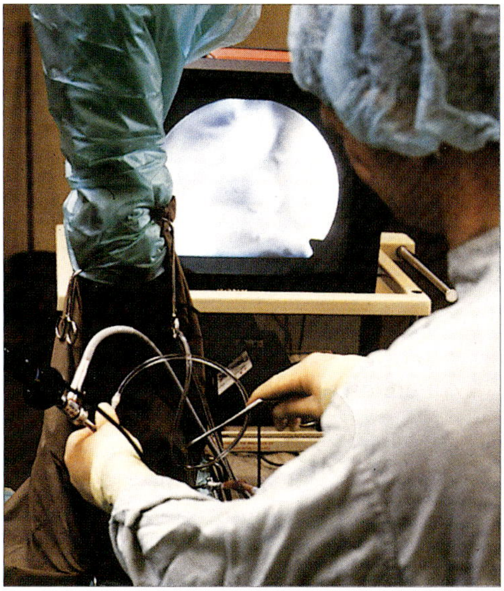

Fig. 6 *Arthroscopy*
A system like a small video endoscope enables the surgeon to see inside a joint, and to operate using tiny power driven tools.

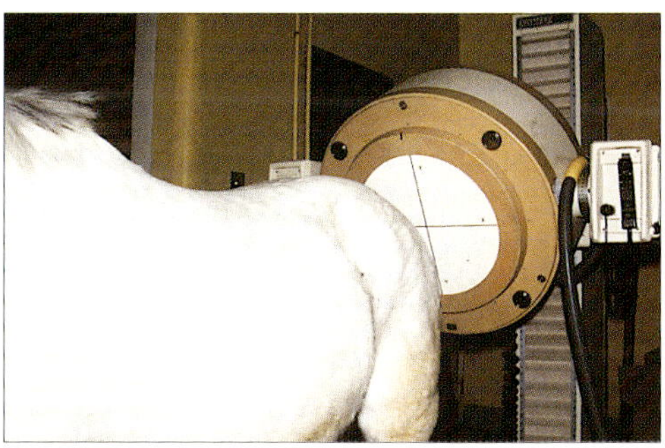

Fig. 7 *Nuclear scintigraphy*
The "camera" counts the radioactive particles emitted from the body, and plots them into a picture which varies in colour or density depending on the amount of radioactivity present.

Nuclear scintigraphy

This technique involves injecting a radioactive substance into the horse's body and then measuring the amount of radioactivity taken up by the various parts of the body. A relative increase in isotopes taken up in one part compared with another means there is more activity in that area than the other *(Fig. 7)*. It is particularly useful as a screening technique to indicate possible areas of inflammation which might be the seat of lameness.

Bacterial and virological culture

We may suspect the presence of bacteria or viruses in a horse, but be unable to see or identify them. In the laboratory, culturing techniques provide ideal conditions for bacterial and viral organisms to multiply until there are enough of them to provide proof of identity tests or to be used in tests to monitor the effectiveness of drugs. Culturing viruses is especially difficult because they grow only inside living cells. Clinical details may enable a veterinarian to make an educated guess as to the identity of an infectious agent which is causing a particular illness. A positive identification after culture in a laboratory may enable us to say definitely that a particular agent is present, and so to plan our efforts to control the infection on appropriate lines.

2: First aid

The healthy horse

Before you are able to assess whether a horse is ill, you must first be fully aware of what is 'normal'. Normally, healthy horses do not:

- *have a nasal discharge*
- *cough more than once or twice at a time*
- *cough when they start work*
- *have loose, unformed droppings*
- *appear lame (even on uneven or hard ground)*
- *leave a normal feed untouched or stand in a field without grazing*
- *have any discharge from their eyes*
- *have any filling, or oedema, of their legs.*

A lame horse is one which, because of pain associated with taking weight on a particular leg, compensates by putting extra weight on the other fore or hind leg. We see this as a nodding of the head when the horse puts extra weight on a foreleg, or as a sinking of the tail and hindquarters when the horse puts the extra weight on a hind leg. Do not make the mistake of thinking that the leg which is hitting the ground when the horse nods, for example, is the lame leg. It is the other foreleg which is painful *(Fig. 8)*.

Lameness can only be evaluated when a horse is being trotted in-hand on a hard surface without a rider. It may not show at all during the walk or canter, and may be masked by the weight and movement of the rider when ridden. Foreleg lameness may also become more apparent by trotting in a small circle. Indeed, some very slight lamenesses may only be detected in this way *(Fig. 9)*. Flexion tests may help confirm the site of a problem by exaggerating the lameness *(Figs. 10 & 11)*.

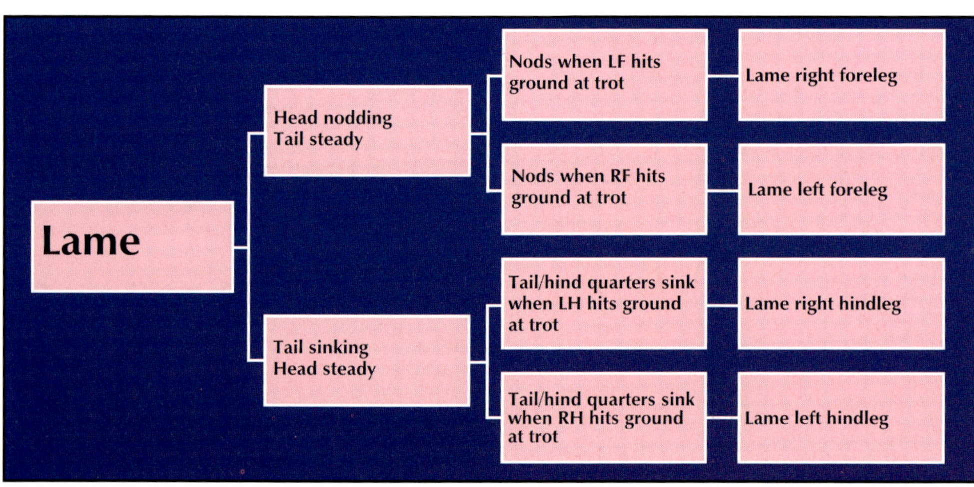

Fig. 8 *Detection of lameness*

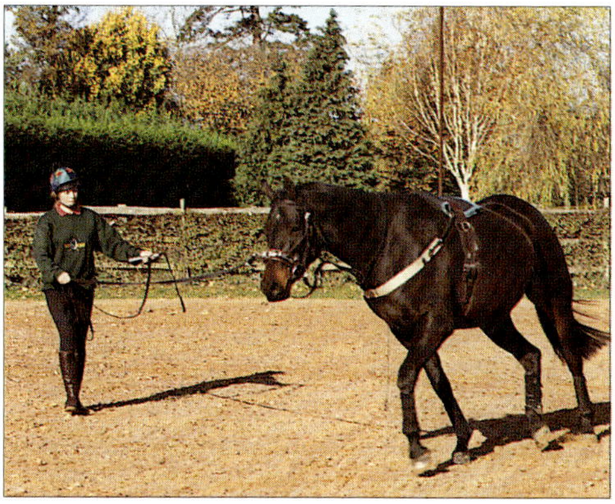

Fig. 9 *Trotting horse in circle – lameness detection test*

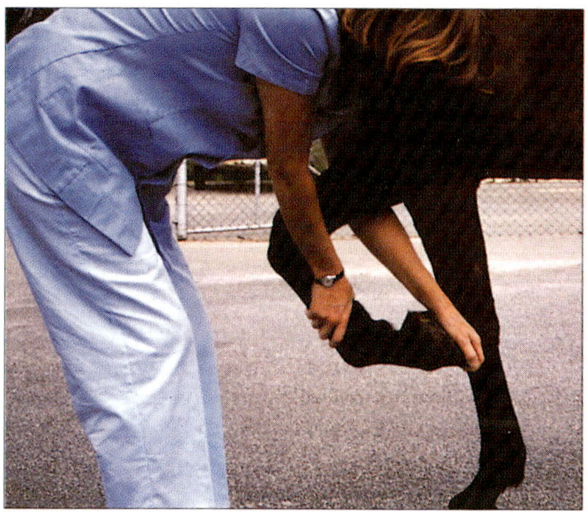

Fig. 10 *Flexion test – fore leg*
The joints are held firmly flexed for at least 30 seconds before the horse is trotted away.

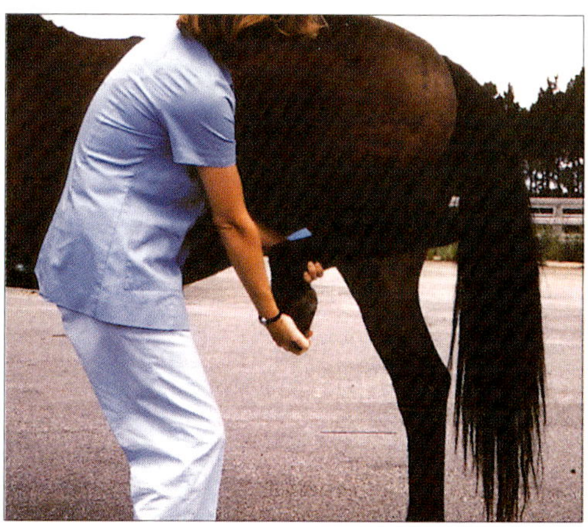

Fig. 11 *Flexion test – hind leg*
This is also known as the spavin test.

Fahrenheit	Centigrade	
99.5	37.5	
100.4	38.0	Normal horse's
101.3	38.5	temperature
102.2	39.0	
103.1	39.5	
104.0	40.0	
104.9	40.5	
105.8	41.0	

Fig. 12 *Comparison of Fahrenheit and Celsius temperatures*

The horse's normal body temperature is 101/101.5°F (38.5°C) *(Fig. 12)*. This is taken by inserting a clinical thermometer with a stubby mercury bulb (not the elongated bulb sometimes found in thermometers for human use) into the horse's rectum. The thermometer should first be held by the end away from the bulb and shaken vigorously in order to ensure that it is not already giving a reading. It should then be inserted for at least half its length, bulb first, and held in place so that if the horse passes some faeces it does not also push out and break the thermometer. The horse will resent the insertion of the thermometer less if the bulb is lubricated with petroleum jelly.

One minute should be allowed before removing the thermometer and reading the temperature. It can take some practice to get used to seeing the column of mercury in the thermometer, and assessing where the end of this column comes in relation to the figure scale. The mercury can only be seen when the stem has been turned to the right angle. If you have difficulty in learning how to do this, buy an electronic thermometer with a digital read-out.

Temperatures below normal are often not significant if the horse appears otherwise healthy. If a horse has recently passed some faeces, for instance, the thermometer may give a low reading because the rectal wall will not have regained its normal temperature. Temperatures above 102°F (38.9°C) are, however, significant. By and large, horses seem to need more provocation to push their temperatures up than do most animals. So when a horse is running a fever it really is significant. In some viral infections the temperature can change very quickly. Do not therefore take your horse's temperature on just one occasion if you are suspicious that there is something wrong – take it every three or four hours. If the resting body temperature reaches 107°F (41.7°C), death is imminent because of damage to the vital internal organs.

The horse's resting heart rate is around 40 to 50 beats per minute. Note that I stress 'resting'. Even the slightest excitement may cause a sharp rise in that figure, so we must interpret fast heart rates carefully. The heart rate can be counted using a stethoscope to listen to the actual heartbeats, or by taking the horse's pulse at the point where an artery crosses over the bottom edge of the lower jaw. It may take some practice to take a horse's pulse, so try doing it while the horse is healthy and it does not matter *(Fig. 13)*.

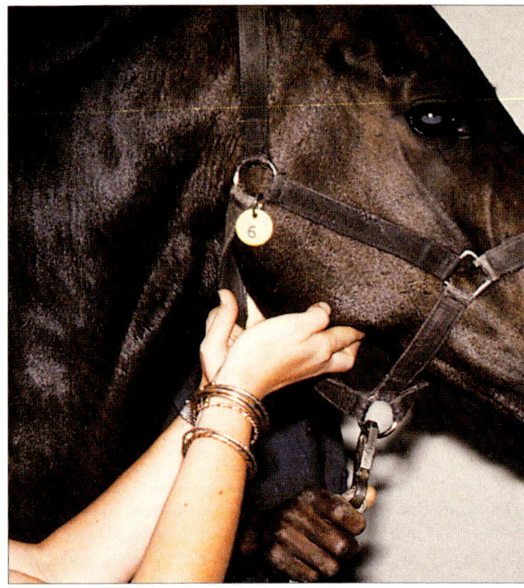

Fig. 13 *Taking a horse's pulse*
The pulse is felt just inside the lower jaw.

When we look at a resting horse in the stable, we can see its chest move as it breathes in and out. The horse's resting respiratory rate is 8 to 16 breaths per minute. A respiratory rate over 20 per minute is usually significant. For both heart rate and respiratory rate, the larger, more placid or fitter the horse, the slower both the heart and respiratory rates will be. When the horse breathes out it should do so in one smooth movement of its rib cage. If there is a momentary break in the middle of this movement, the horse may be said to be broken-winded. The hesitation comes from the need to use conscious muscular effort to empty the rest of the air out of the lungs when the normal elastic recoil has failed to do so. When such effort is necessary the muscular walls of the abdomen can also be seen to move in and out. In a healthy horse the pulse rate is usually three times the respiratory rate, even when both have been dramatically increased by exercise. If the ratio approaches 1:1, then there may be a serious respiratory problem.

So far I have discussed some of the indicators of health and distress, some of which can be seen literally over the stable door.

Stepping into the stable we can actually touch the horse. Its skin should be supple and elastic. If we pick up a fold of skin over the neck or shoulder, it should flatten again as soon as we let it go. If the fold remains, or collapses only slowly, the horse is probably dehydrated. If a horse is stabled all the time its coat might become very dusty, but otherwise a healthy horse has a bright shiny coat during the summer, even if it has not been groomed. The long, thick winter coat should be even all over, without any evidence that parts of it have been rubbed or nibbled away.

During grooming we have the opportunity to feel all over the body for any swellings or painful areas. It is important that the hooves are picked out regularly, especially along the clefts on either side of the frog. A healthy hoof does not smell offensive. Nor is there any foul-smelling black liquid in the frog clefts, indicative of a thrush infection.

Horses tend to be creatures of habit, and so any deviation from their normal behaviour should be noted. In particular we should be aware whether a horse normally eats its food quickly or over a long period *(Fig. 14)*. A horse will normally pass between two and four piles of faeces when stabled overnight. These should be firm in consistency, although they may be accompanied by some brown fluid. When a horse is turned out on growing grass for at least part of the day, its droppings may be soft and more like a cow's dung pat. They should not, however, be watery. Diarrhoea is rare in the horse.

Horses are creatures of habit in regard to their urination. Some will wait until they have eaten before they pass urine, others hardly ever pass urine in the stable but do so as soon as they are taken outside. We should know what an individual horse's habit is. The character of the urine is not important because there is so much variation even in healthy horses.

Many horses have been conditioned by their owners into drinking only at certain times. In the wild, horses drink around the time they are feeding, but traditionally some people prevent their horses from doing so for fear that the cold water may trigger off a digestive upset. The amount of water consumed naturally varies with size and with the environmental temperature. A stabled horse receiving only dry food may drink between four and seventeen gallons.

Owners should know whether their horse normally lies down in the stable, and how much time it spends looking over the stable door. Any variation in this sort of behaviour may indicate that the horse is not feeling well in some way.

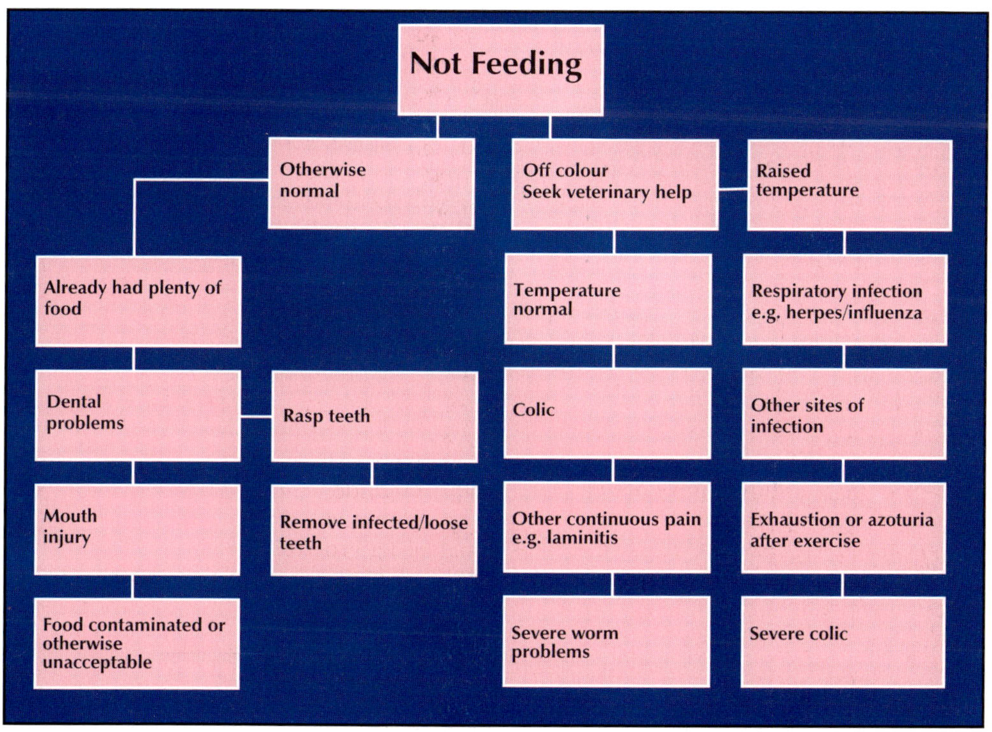

Fig. 14 *Flow chart examining the causes of loss of appetite*

The first aid kit

This is a very important part of the armoury in the fight against disease. In many cases the first aid treatment carried out by the horse owner before the veterinarian arrives on the scene can have a dramatic effect on the eventual outcome. A first aid kit is only of use if it is available at the time and place of the injury; it is of no value at home if the horse cuts itself at a show. It is therefore important to have a first aid kit in the horsebox or trailer as well. Of course, injuries can occur when hacking many miles away from either stable or horsebox. You should therefore also consider carrying a very small, simple kit in your pocket whenever you are riding any distance.

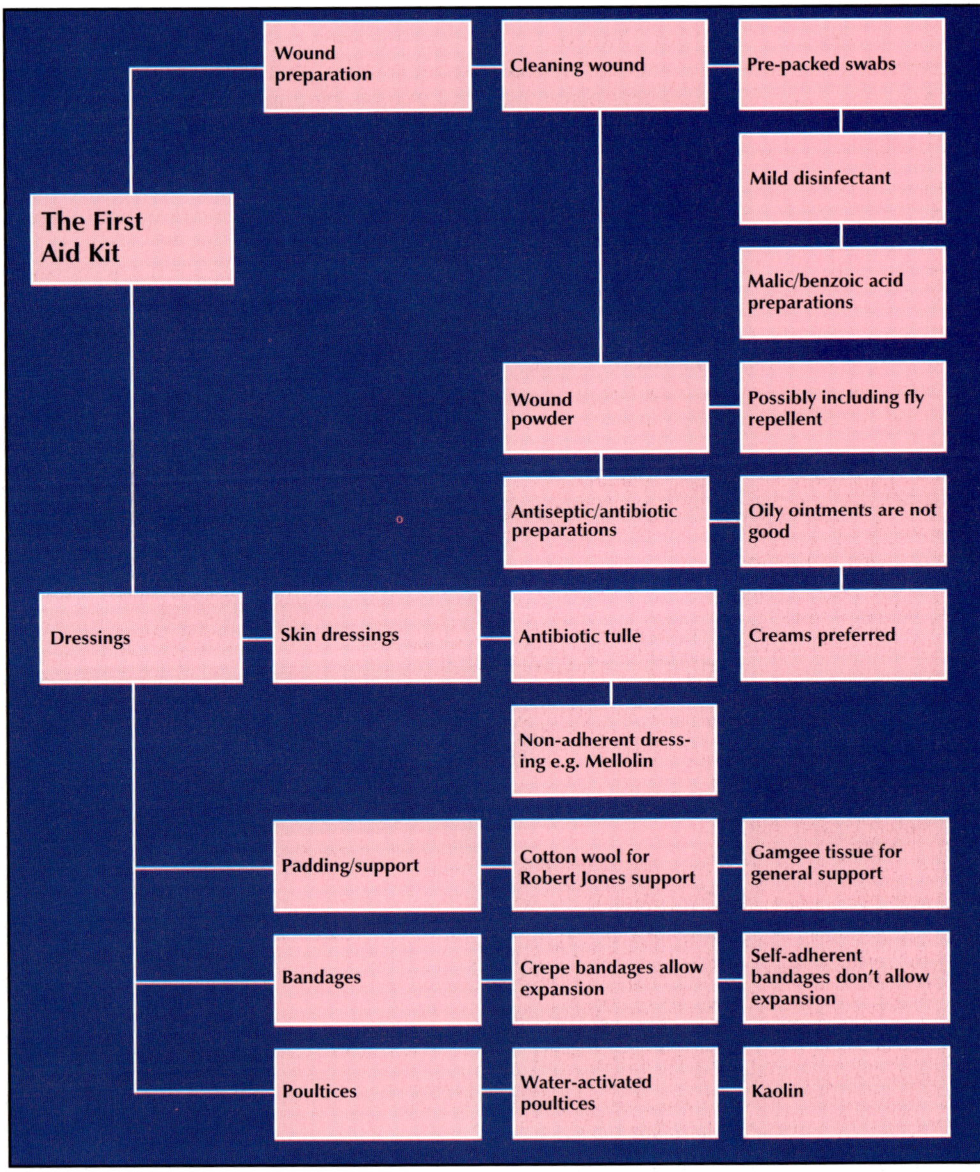

Fig. 15 *The first aid kit* The equipment you should include for different situations.

Much of the contents of a first aid kit are for dealing with wounds *(Fig. 15)*. There should always be something to clean the wound, such as cotton swabs and antiseptic solution, which can be added to the water used for cleaning. Antiseptic-impregnated swabs are also available for this purpose. They have the advantage that they make you independent of a clean water supply. Don't forget that washing a wound with dirty water will make things worse rather than better because it introduces yet another source of infection. Many horse owners place too much reliance on washing wounds: it is far more important to stop a haemorrhage than to wash everything surgically clean, and the bleeding will not stop while you are continually washing away the clot which is trying to form *(Fig. 16)*.

It is extremely unlikely that owners will ever have to deal with a horse with a cut artery, because superficial arteries are relatively small vessels with a tough wall. Arterial blood is bright red and will spurt several feet into the air away from the wound. A horse can die within minutes of cutting a major artery, so there is no time to summon help or fetch a first aid kit.

Pressure must be applied at once to the source of the bleeding, using a pad made from an item of clothing, for example. If there is nobody else to summon veterinary help, pressure must be applied for at least 30 to 40 minutes before checking whether a clot has formed. Fortunately, most bleeding is either continual oozing from small capillary vessels or more forceful venous bleeding. When assessing how much blood a horse has lost, remember that a large horse can literally lose bucketsful without any serious effects.

The best way to stop a haemorrhage of any kind is to apply firm pressure directly to the wound, and to continue to do so until the bleeding has stopped. This can take just a couple of minutes, but even with some larger veins it may take up to an hour. The first aid kit must include some clean pads for placing over such

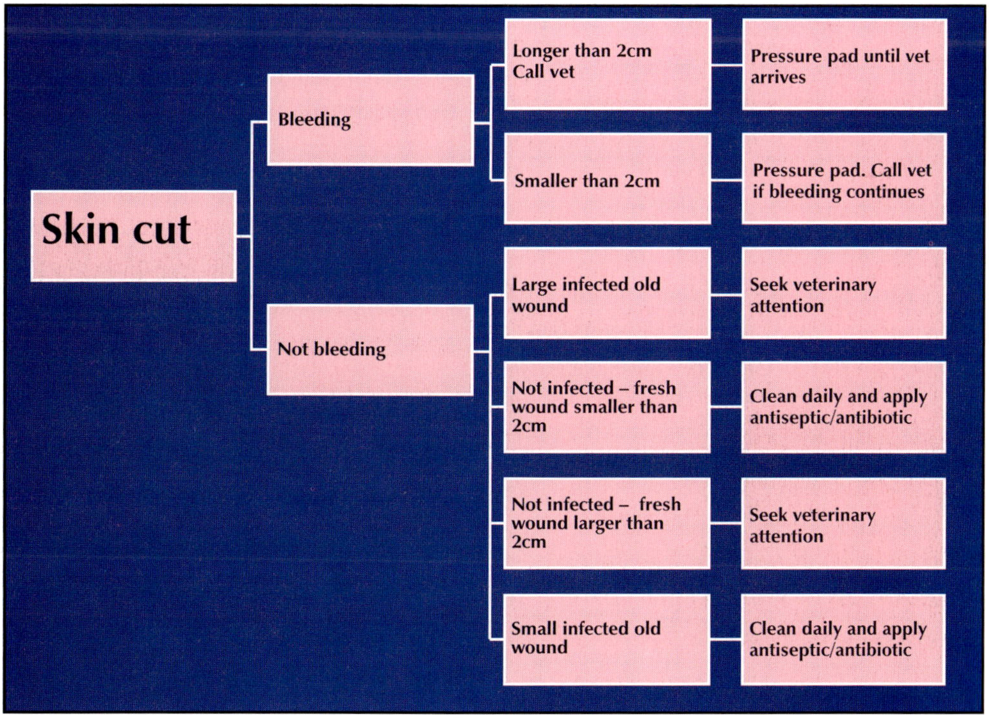

Fig. 16 *A guide to the treatment of skin wounds*

wounds. These must not stick to the wound, otherwise their removal may start the bleeding again *(Fig. 17)*.

Never use cotton swabs for this purpose. They stick both to the wound and the surrounding bloody skin. Non-stick tulle impregnated with an antibiotic makes an ideal wound dressing. When infection is not suspected, lint pads, which incorporate a sheet of plastic film, can be useful because the blood or tissue fluids pass through the plastic film (which is placed directly in contact with the wound) and are absorbed by the lint.

Gamgee tissue is an important part of every first aid kit. It can be used to make a pad which is then bandaged or (if the wound involves a part of the horse's body which cannot readily be bandaged) held firmly over a wound until the bleeding stops. In almost every respect Gamgee tissue is easier to use than cotton swabs. It can also be used as part of a 'Robert Jones' bandage *(Fig. 18)*. This is a means of temporarily immobilising a horse's leg when you suspect a fracture or some other serious injury. The basic idea is to apply a thick enough layer of padding to

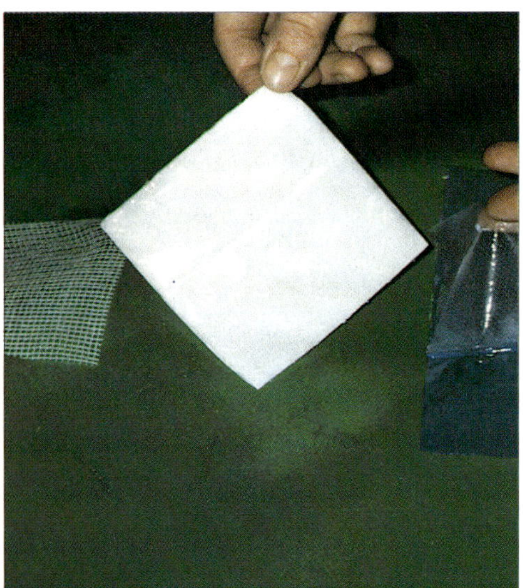

Fig. 17 *A selection of non-stick dressings – tulle, kaolin and hydrogel*

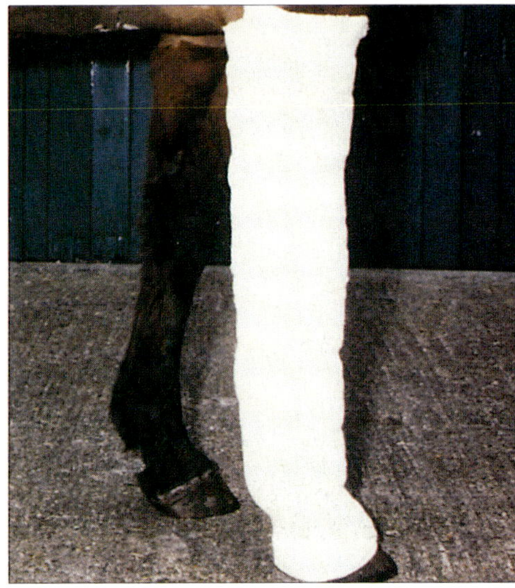

Fig. 18 *A Robert Jones bandage*

prevent any bending of the leg. This requires at least four layers of Gamgee, plus bandages. As the dressing must extend from the hoof to the elbow or stifle, several large rolls of Gamgee must be kept in the first aid kit. This is, of course, very bulky but if it saves a horse's active life that does not matter.

Which bandages should you include in a first aid kit? Although cheap to buy, cotton open weave bandages have no place here. They are dangerous, because when they are applied tightly enough to hold a dressing in place, their edges will dig into the skin and cause new problems. In addition they neither adapt to the contours of the leg nor provide any 'give' if the leg swells after bandaging. Any proprietary horse first aid kit containing open weave bandages should be discarded on the grounds that if the manufacturer can make such an elementary mistake, then the rest of the contents must be suspect.

Crepe bandages, usually 5cm (2in) wide, are good as they have some elasticity and can mould to the contours of the leg. Self-adherent or cohesive bandages are more expensive but are also useful. They mould well to the shape of the part being bandaged, but they do not allow the

Figs. 19 - 23 *Applying a dressing to a horse's leg – Step by step*

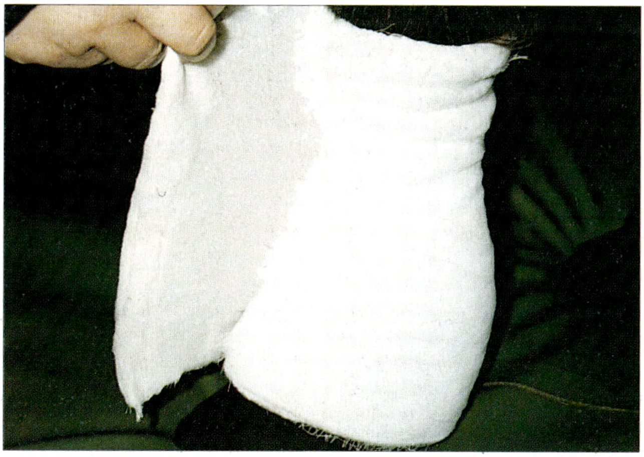

Fig. 19 Gamgee is wrapped around the leg.

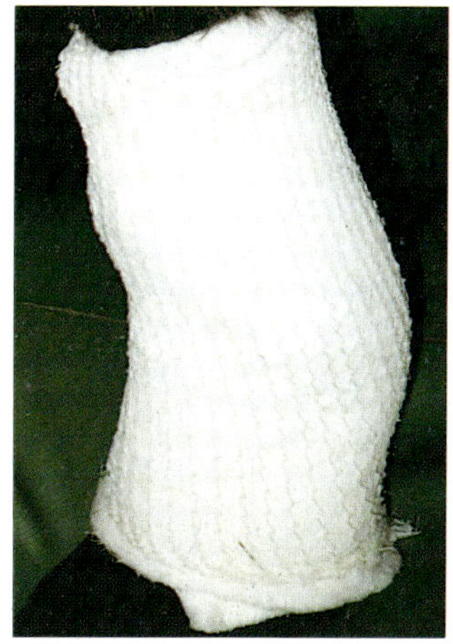

Fig. 20 Gamgee in place.

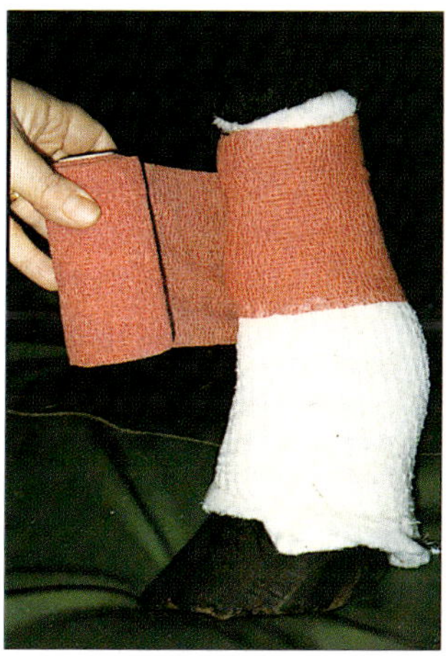

Fig. 21 Start bandaging at the top, working from left to right.

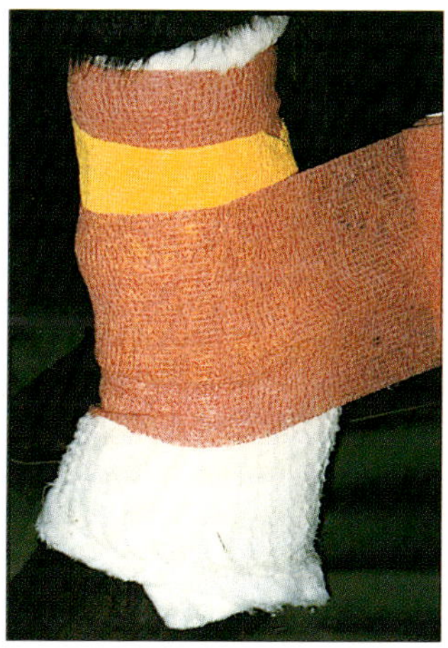

Fig. 22 Each layer of bandage overlaps its predecessor by approximately 50%.

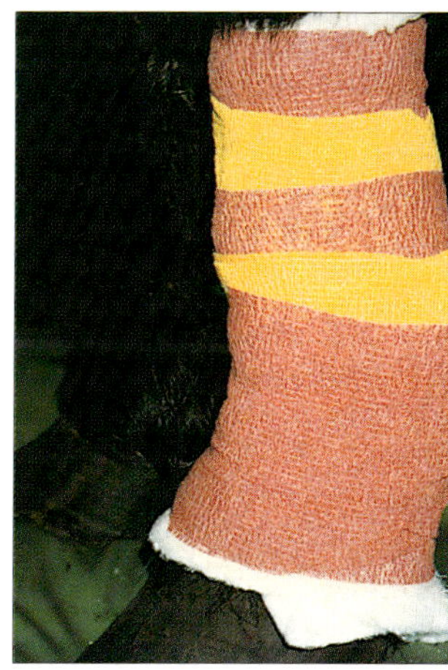

Fig. 23 The finished product.

injured part to swell any further, because once a second layer has been applied they cannot stretch. A useful point is that if a horse fidgets while someone is bandaging say, a leg with a self-adherent bandage and it is jerked out of their hand, it will not unroll all over the floor in the way that other bandages do.

It is a regrettable fact of life that a horse's legs are designed to make bandaging as problematic as possible. Applying the bandage itself is not too difficult. You start at the top, leaving about 2.5cm (1in) of Gamgee above the first layer of bandage *(Figs. 19-23)*. If you are right-handed the roll of bandage runs to your right, with the unrolling part flat on the leg. The second round should be directly on top of the first, in order to anchor it. After that each layer overlaps approximately half of its predecessor. The first difficulty is in getting the tension right. Too tight and you impede the circulation and, especially down the cannon, possibly damage the

Figs. 24 - 26 *Bandaging a hock*

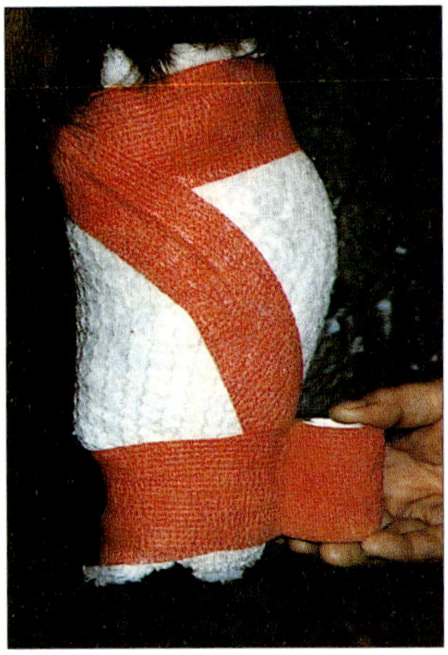

Fig. 24 Anchor the bandage at the top and then go diagonally down to the bottom of the dressing.

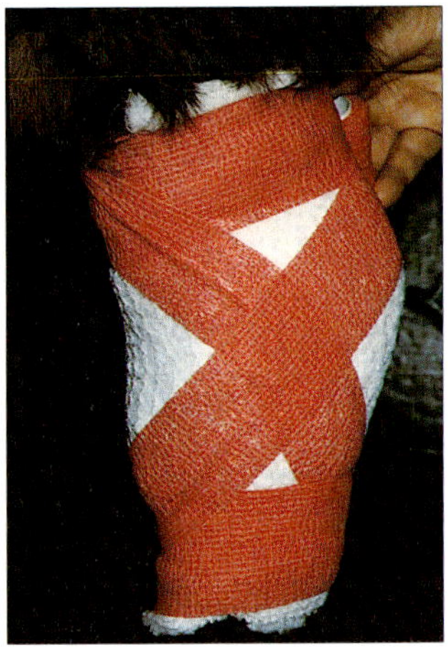

Fig. 25 Then go diagonally up to the top, crossing the earlier bandage.

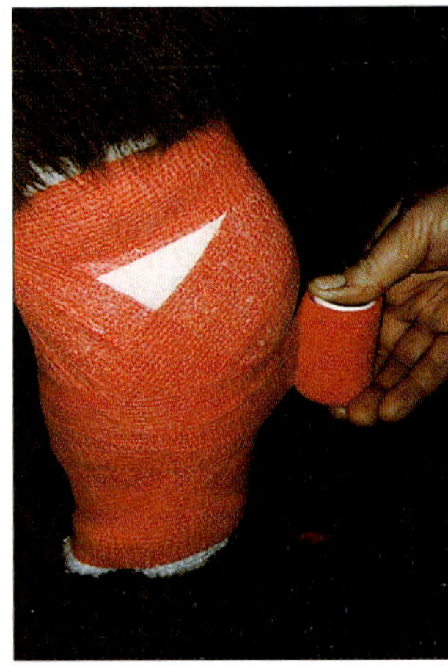

Fig. 26 The almost finished bandage.

underlying tendons. Too loose and the dressing ends up around the horse's foot. You can prevent the dressing from slipping either by anchoring the top and bottom with a single round of stretch adhesive dressing, or by putting a thick layer of separate dressing from the foot up to the bottom of the dressing, thus providing a ledge on which the real dressing rests. Hocks require figure of eight bandaging *(Figs. 24-26)*. Feet also pose awkward problems *(Figs. 27-29)*.

The first aid kit should include some form of poultice dressing. The aim of poulticing is to draw infected material out of a wound. Kaolin, for example, can be heated up in its tin by placing it in a pan of boiling water. When hot, the kaolin paste should be smeared on to a piece of aluminium foil and then applied to the affected area so that the foil reflects the heat back on to the leg.

Alternatively, a thin flat parcel of kaolin can be made using foil with the edges folded several times; this is then heated as above. This does not take as long, and it may be sufficient to place the poultice in a dish, pour boiling water over it, and leave it to stand for a minute or two. The temperature of any poultice must not be hotter than you can stand on your own skin.

Water-activated poultices (e.g. Animalintex in the UK) are a form of impregnated Gamgee which become effective after soaking in warm water *(Fig. 30)*. The dressing is then drained briefly *(Fig. 31)* and put in position, with a sheet of waterproof polythene between the wet poultice and the bandages which hold it in place. In the past poultices were also made by pouring boiling water over bran or stale bread, and mixing the result into a paste which was then applied. This can still be useful if for some reason there is no proper poultice available, but such a poultice does not retain its heat very well and has little 'drawing' power.

Poultices do not remain active forever. When they have cooled down to body temperature they have little effect and need to be replaced at least two or three times per day. It is important to note that wounds should never be poulticed for more than 48 hours unless on veterinary advice. Poulticing softens the skin and may prevent wound edges from healing.

Poultices on the leg can be bandaged

Figs. 27 - 29 *Bandaging a foot*

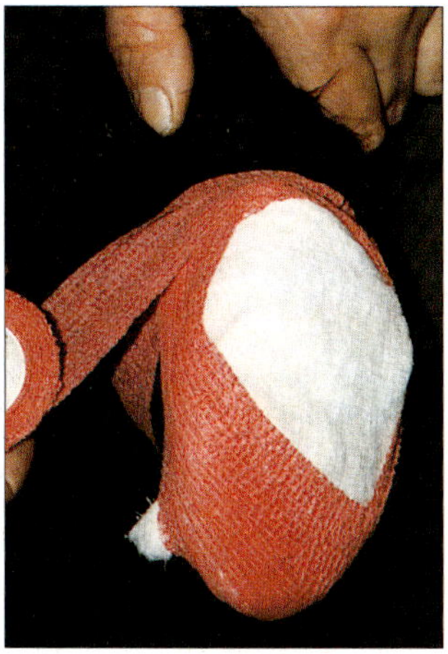

Fig. 27 First bandage around the hoof wall, then include the toe.

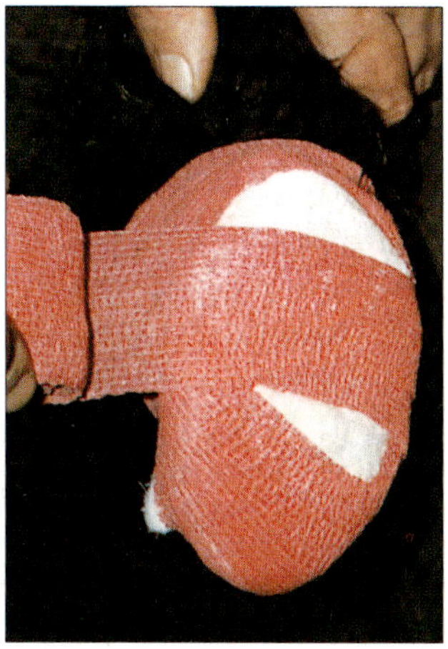

Fig. 28 Bandage across the bottom of the foot and around the front of the hoof.

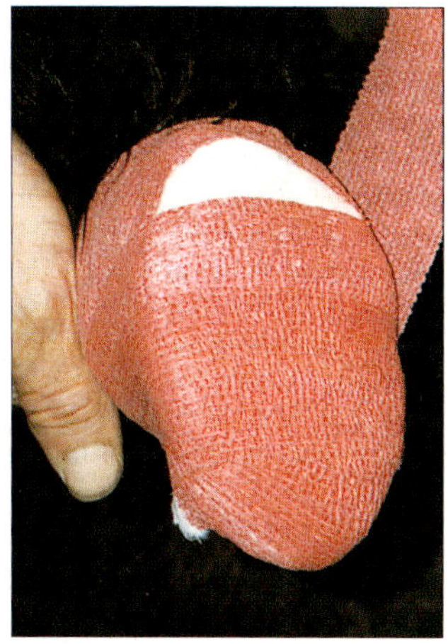

Fig. 29 The almost finished bandage.

in place like any other dressing. When puncture wounds of the foot need poulticing, however, it can be more difficult to keep the poultice in place. Purpose-made plastic poultice boots and shoes make the task easier. In the absence of such aids the poultice will need to be strapped to the foot with adhesive stretch tape, and then the whole foot enclosed in a thick plastic sack to protect it from damp bedding.

The local blood supply is increased by poultices. They are not therefore effective in reducing the swelling associated with physical injuries such as sprains, where there is no wound. In this situation the application of cool materials is the best treatment as it will constrict the blood vessels supplying the area. Gentle hosing with cold water provides a source of relief.

Unfortunately hosing is only effective as a source of cooling while it is being carried out, so it is time-consuming. Special dressings are available that can be applied to the leg and then attached to a

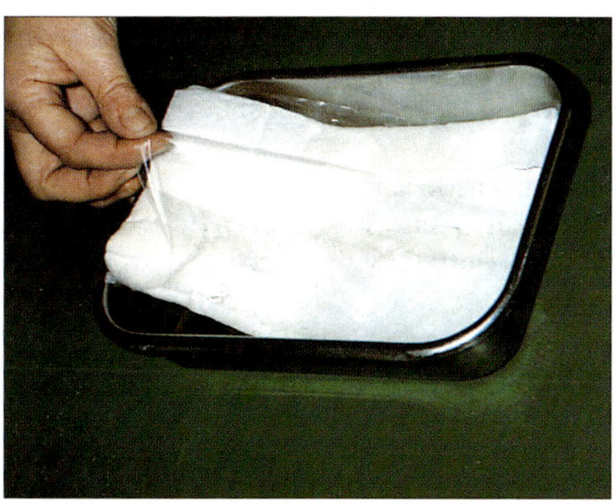

Fig. 30 *Soak the water-activated poultice in warm water, plastic side uppermost*

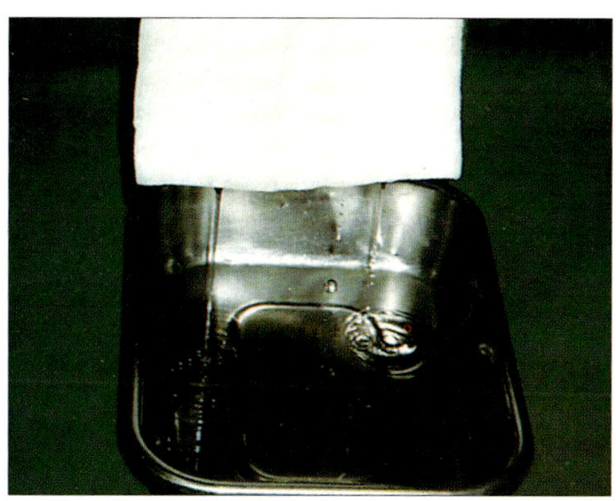

Fig. 31 *Drain the poultice before applying to the horse*

hosepipe, so that the leg can be hosed without having to actually hold the pipe all the time. For placid horses this can be very useful, although drainage of the water can be a problem.

Kaolin also retains cold as well as heat. It can be chilled in a fridge, either in its tin or as a foil parcel in the way already described for a hot poultice. Ice packs made from ice cubes or even a bag of frozen peas can be effective in cooling a leg. A more long-lasting effect can be obtained from commercial gel packs which can be re-chilled in a freezer. Ideally you should always have one ready chilled, as treatment can be delayed for a couple of hours if you have to start from scratch.

The 'Bonner' bandage is a special bandage which is soaked in water and then frozen. It remains flexible enough when frozen to be applied to the leg. Because it provides freezing cold all around the leg it should not be left in place for more than an hour at a time. In any event, ice preparations should never be placed in direct contact with the skin. A thin layer of bandage of some kind should always separate the two. There are proprietary gels which cool by chemical action. Care must be taken in using them where there are any skin wounds as their chemicals may further inflame the wound.

The final component of the first aid kit is some form of wound dressing. This may take the form of an aerosol. It is unfortunate that some horses will not tolerate the noise of an aerosol, because it provides a very good means of applying antibiotics to wounds. Alternatively, there are many different wound powders available. The important thing is not to apply them too enthusiastically. A thick layer of powder over an open wound usually results in a dry top scab protecting a wet lower layer of exhausted powder mixed with infected pus. Ointments and oils should never be applied to wounds without specific veterinary instructions. They irritate the deeper tissues, form a barrier between wound edges to prevent healing, and may make it unsafe for the veterinarian to stitch the wound if it proves necessary.

Owners must never forget that first aid means just that. When 'second aid' is required they must seek veterinary assistance. Sometimes it may be difficult to know when this is warranted, and when it isn't. The following circumstances may indicate when veterinary help should be sought:

- *If the horse's temperature is over 102°F (38.9°C).*
- *If the horse's resting respiratory rate is over 20 per minute.*
- *If the horse's resting heart rate is increasing from its normal rate.*
- *If the horse has mild colic for more than 30 minutes or has short recurring bouts of mild colic.*
- *If the horse has acute colic and is throwing itself to the ground.*
- *If the horse is acutely lame and not bearing weight on a leg.*
- *If a horse is lame, however slightly, for more than 24 hours.*
- *If a wound continues to bleed despite pressure bandaging.*
- *If a wound is longer than 2.5cm (1in)*
- *If a horse is recumbent from any cause and unwilling to rise.*

There are some vital rules that are often forgotten in advice on first aid. They concern what should be done when the emergency is first discovered. If a horse is found standing on three legs, unwilling to let the other leg even touch the ground, and evades your attempts to catch it, it should be left alone. There will be plenty of time to catch the horse when veterinary help has been summoned. If there is a fractured bone in the leg then the less movement from the horse, the better. When help is on its way (and the first aid kit has been collected), catch the horse and apply a Robert Jones bandage.

Sometimes a horse appears at first to be

anxious to avoid putting weight on a particular leg, but when it starts to move it becomes clear that it will put its toe to the ground and put some weight on it. Rather than walk the horse back to the stable you should leave it where it is until it has been properly examined by the veterinarian. There is little chance that the horse will make its situation worse by standing still, no matter what the problem is, but there is a good chance that even a short walk will make a major orthopaedic problem worse.

I have already suggested that if a horse is lying down and unwilling to rise then veterinary help is essential. Perhaps this needs some clarification. Horses with certain types of colic will continue to lie down when approached by their owner. If, however, they are firmly roused they can and will stand up. A horse which has injured its back severely, on the other hand, cannot get up even if it tries.

I advise that one really strenuous attempt is made to stimulate a horse to stand up. Once this has been tried and has failed, then do not attempt it again until veterinary help arrives. In the meantime, the horse should be protected from the elements, especially cold and moisture. It should also be protected from any other horses in the field, because by their curiosity they can cause the horse to damage itself further as it tries to avoid their attention.

Horse owners should make sure that they know their veterinarian well, and that he or she knows them. They should check which are the best times to contact the clinic for advice, and which telephone number to use. Evenings and weekends are usually kept for emergencies only. Sometimes a different telephone number should be used in such circumstances. All the relevant telephone numbers should be clearly displayed in the tack room and in the first aid kits. Owners should also make sure that they know exactly where the clinic is in case they need to take their horse there in an emergency.

Pain

Pain can affect a horse in various ways. Acute local pain in the foot may be easy to recognise because the horse will not put any weight on that foot, and will hold it off the ground. Acute abdominal pain, or colic, may cause the horse to throw itself to the ground and roll violently. The following conditions indicate that the horse may be in pain:

- *Increase in the horse's pulse rate.*
- *Increase in the horse's respiratory rate.*
- *Increase in the horse's temperature even when no infection is present.*
- *Sweating when the horse has not been exercising.*
- *Apprehension, which shows in an over-alert response to the environment and any movement the owner makes.*
- *Lack of interest in food.*
- *General dullness or other change in temperament.*

There are no home remedies for relieving a horse's pain. If a horse is in pain then veterinary assistance should be sought.

3: Planning for health

Buying a horse

'Let the buyer beware' is appropriate advice for anyone buying a horse. Nothing brings out the worst in people (including friends and relations) more than negotiating the sale of a horse or a car. The first step in buying a horse is to decide what you want the the horse to do. You should then stick to this job description, no matter how much someone tries to tell you that what you need is a racehorse or a mountain pony (which they just happen to have for sale).

Then you can go and find a horse, at the price you can afford, which does that job. If looking pretty is not part of that job description, you should not include it in your screening criteria. Never fall into the temptation of assuming that after purchase you will be able to do things with the horse that its present owner has failed to do. If a horse cannot jump four and a half feet at eight years old, it is more likely to be due to lack of ability than an incompetent past owner.

Veterinary aspects of the purchase should be the final consideration. Only when you are sure that you want to buy the horse in all other respects should you consider calling in the veterinarian for advice. This means that you may occasionally be disappointed, but you are less likely to acquire a horse that you did not really want just because it sailed through a veterinary examination. Once you have decided on the horse you want, it is important that you have it examined by an experienced veterinarian. You can do some of the tests yourself: these will be described in due course. But there is no substitute for an opinion by a qualified and objective person.

In most countries, the form of the veterinary examination is laid down by a regulatory body or association (see appendix page 172). The aim is to reach a decision over whether to recommend purchase of the horse for a specific purpose or not. Although veterinarians no longer pronounce a horse 'sound', the implied meaning of that word is still there. In other words, the veterinarian is saying that it is reasonable to buy the horse because there are no problems detected which might now or in the near future affect its ability to carry out that specified work.

The choice of veterinarian is the purchaser's. If their usual veterinarian also acts for the vendor, he or she can still examine the horse on their behalf as long as the vendor agrees to disclose everything they know about the horse. This means that the purchaser gets the past history as well as a present appraisal. If distance prevents their usual veterinarian from examining the horse, he or she will usually be able to suggest a local experienced colleague. It may be better to ask a good horse veterinarian to travel a little distance to see the horse rather than use the nearest one who only treats horses occasionally.

The examination consists of several parts *(Fig. 32)*. The first stage of the purchase examination is to examine the horse in the stable. The external appearance of each part of the horse's body is examined and any lumps and bumps noted. The heart and lungs are listened to carefully, although slight heart abnormalities at rest are often of no significance. The legs and feet undergo close scrutiny, which includes pressure around the hoof. It is surprising how often this stage of the examination reveals abnormalities of which the owner was completely unaware.

Veterinary examination for purchase
Stage 1) Preliminary examination in stable
Stage 2) Trotting up
Stage 3) Strenuous exercise
Stage 4) Rest period
Stage 5) Second trot and foot examination

Fig. 32 *Veterinary examination for purchase*

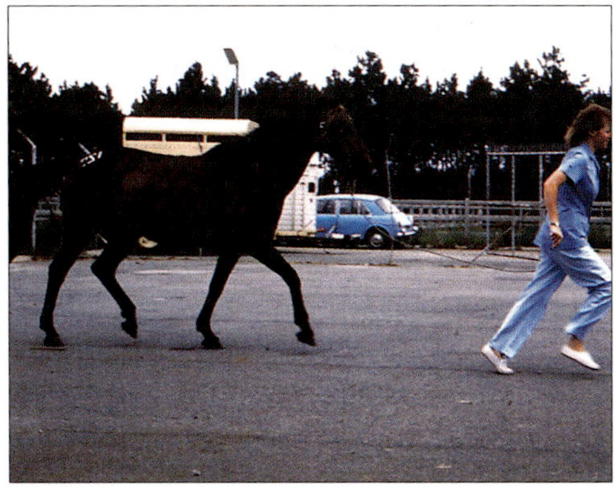

Fig. 33 *Trotting horse up*

The horse is then brought out on a head collar and rope – that is, under minimal restriction. It is examined at the walk and the trot *(Fig. 33)*. Some veterinarians include trotting in a small circle, some include flexion tests which involve holding the lower joints of the leg tightly flexed for 30 seconds or more and then trotting the horse straight off. When this is carried out on the hind legs it is often called the spavin test. Normally, horses do not trot lame for more than one or two strides after a flexion test. The horse is also observed going backwards and turning on the spot.

The third part of the examination is a period of strenuous exercise under saddle. The extent of the exercise will bear some relationship to the proposed workload. In any case it must be sufficient to markedly raise the heart rate. Lunging exercise is only really a valid alternative in young, unbroken horses. Absence of a rider or of somewhere to canter are not sufficient excuses to justify omitting this section. As soon as the exercise is stopped the veterinarian listens to the heart and lungs. The former slows down very quickly, so the examination must not be delayed.

In order to give muscles and joints a chance to stiffen up, the horse is then rested. During this time the eyes are usually examined in a darkened stable using an ophthalmoscope. Then the horse is trotted again in hand to check for lameness. Finally, the identification of the horse is described on the official form.

If the veterinarian finds something during the examination which prevents them from recommending purchase, they may cut the examination short. Whatever happens, he or she must report to the purchaser, not to the person selling the horse. The veterinarian does not investigate the problem, which is the responsibility of the vendor and his veterinarian.

So, for example, if a horse is lame, it fails the examination. But the examining veterinarian does not go on to nerve blocks and so on in an attempt to find the cause. Indeed, strictly speaking the vendor should not even be told whether purchase will be recommended or not. The buyer should be the one to hear and assess that information.

There are other aspects that can be included in a purchase examination. Increasingly, a blood sample is taken and stored in case there is any possibility of the horse having been under the influence of pain-killing drugs prior to the sale. An endoscopic examination may be included specifically to determine whether laryngeal hemiplegia (see page 49) is present. Somewhat controversially, X-rays may be taken of the feet and/or joints. X-rays may reveal a problem, but may also disclose minor bony changes which do not cause any clinical symptoms. They may show that there is no abnormality present at the time which is good, but the horse might still be crippled with navicular disease (see page 161) seven or eight weeks later. The consensus of opinion in the UK is that when a thorough purchase examination has been carried out, X-rays do not add anything unless there is a specific lesion to be evaluated. X-ray findings must not be equated with painful lesions that will cause lameness: many horses have X-ray abnormalities but are not lame.

While you, as purchaser, will be relying on your own veterinary examination, you should still obtain as comprehensive a warranty from the vendor as possible. In particular you should ask the vendor to certify, preferably in writing or in front of a witness, that the horse is free from stable vices (see e.g. crib biting and windsucking, Chapter 5).

These are not included in a veterinary report because they will not usually be apparent during the examination. The horse tends to indulge in such vices when it is quiet and relaxed. It is also reasonable to ask the vendor to warrant that the horse is sound. He is then sharing some of the responsibility with the veterinary advisor on whose professional advice you will rely, but against whom you have a redress if that advice is negligent.

It is usually best to get the horse home as soon as possible after purchase. Accidents can happen at any time, and it is very difficult to assign responsibility if a horse is injured or falls ill after the purchase has been completed but while still in the vendor's care.

On arrival the new horse should be dewormed and kept stabled for 24 hours. This ensures that if it has a worm burden it does not contaminate the pasture. If this is not possible, turn it out in the smallest possible area and remove all the droppings for the first couple of days.

If other horses are on the premises, there is the risk that the new horse, while appearing to be healthy, will introduce infections such as those caused by respiratory viruses. The new horse may be immune to a particular strain of virus that the other horses may not have been in contact with. Ideally, do not stable the new horse with the other horses for the first week. Isolation will also protect the new horse from any infections that the other horses may have.

With the excitement of a new purchase there is a tendency to overwork the newcomer. Remember that people avoid working horses hard once they have decided to sell them, for fear of bringing on injuries. Purchasers should therefore treat a new horse as if it has just been rested, and gradually build up its work. All too often, horses go lame six to eight weeks after a change of stables because of a change in their exercise pattern. By gradually establishing a new exercise regime it should be possible to prevent this happening.

Horse insurance

A horse of any size represents a considerable financial investment. Anyone selling a horse ought perhaps to be obliged to give the purchaser one of those investment warnings: 'The value of this horse may go up and down depending on circumstances'. An increasing number of owners attempt to safeguard their investment by taking out an insurance policy, but it is important to understand what policies are available and what cover they provide. There are four main elements to horse insurance—cover against death, immediate slaughter on humane grounds, permanent loss of use and veterinary fees. Cover may differ from country to country.

Such policies start with the assumption that the horse is perfectly healthy at commencement. As far as the insurance company is concerned, this does not mean that the owner thought that the horse was normal, but that it actually was normal. If a disease becomes apparent in the early days of the policy and it can be shown to have been present before the policy started the policy will be void, even though the horse had not shown any clinical symptoms when the policy was taken out. For example, a horse might go lame a fortnight after purchase and on X-ray be found to have navicular disease. Even if the horse was vetted at purchase and sound at the inception of the policy, the policy will still be void. Insurance policies relate to disease conditions, not clinical symptoms.

If a horse is not perfectly sound this does not mean that the owner will not be able to insure it. The problem may pose no extra risk for the type of policy they require. A skin problem, for example, would not normally increase the risk of a horse dying in the field. Alternatively, the insurance company may be perfectly willing to insure the horse as long as the particular known problem is excluded from the policy *(Fig. 34)*.

A piece of advice: some insurance companies frame the wording of such exclusion clauses very badly. This is often because the wording is devised by a clerk in an office who has no real knowledge of veterinary matters. Almost always, such companies exclude more then they should. The worst example of this I have come across related to a minor problem of the front legs, but the exclusion was placed on 'the front of the horse'. I dreaded the horse being cut on its body and the owner needing to prove where the front end stopped and the back end started. It is often worthwhile checking with your veterinary advisor whether the proposed exclusion is reasonable before you accept it. Once you have accepted it, you must abide by the consequences.

It sometimes happens that an owner has a horse vetted at purchase and the veterinarian recommends purchase, but when the insurance company sees the veterinary report it insists on excluding one or more conditions. This is not really a reflection on the veterinarian, rather it is a reflection of a different viewpoint. An insurance company may end up insuring the horse for many years, during which time it is used for a variety of activities which might not have been originally envisaged. So inevitably the insurance company takes a reasonably strict point of view. It obviously does not want anyone to think that it is safe to 'take a chance' on a horse on the grounds that if the gamble does not come off, the insurance company will pick up the bill.

Making an insurance claim

1) Notify the insurers at the onset. Do not wait until you are sending off the claim form.
2) Make sure that your veterinarian knows (a) the horse is insured (b) what type of cover you have.
3) If claiming for veterinary fees, send detailed invoices with the claims.
4) If making a loss of use claim, send copies of any second opinion or laboratory reports.
5) If making a loss of use claim, check with your veterinarian that there are no other forms of treatment that could be tried.
6) Do not make decisions on economic grounds alone without involving the insurers.
7) Do not put down an insured horse without first consulting the insurance company, unless it is an emergency decision outside office hours.
8) Your policy will probably require you to have a post mortem examination carried out at your expense if your horse is put down.

Fig. 34 *Making an insurance claim*

When a horse is insured against death, it means death from natural causes or unnatural causes such as a lightning strike or a car accident. The point is that its end is not hastened by man. Usually death cover is linked with cover against the horse needing immediate destruction on humane grounds. The wording of these policies is often misunderstood. For a valid claim the following criteria need to be satisfied:

- *The horse must require immediate destruction.*
- *The horse must be suffering excessive pain which cannot be relieved in any way.*
- *There is no prospect of successful treatment.*

This policy does not allow the horse to be put down simply because it is in pain; it has to be very acute pain that cannot be controlled by painkillers. The policy does not allow the horse to be put down just because it has an incurable condition; it has to also be in acute pain. Hence that critical word 'immediate'. If the decision has been taken to delay euthanasia for several days (or even longer) after the problem appears, it is probable that a claim under this policy will not be valid.

I must stress that insurance companies cannot stop owners putting a horse down if they want to do so; on the other hand, if a horse has been put down it does not automatically mean that they will meet a claim. There are certain conditions which will almost always constitute a valid claim for immediate slaughter on humane grounds. These include fractures of the main leg bones above the knee or hock, compound fractures (where the bone has penetrated the skin), certain very acute colic problems and complete rupture of the flexor tendons.

It is a condition of the policy that if at all possible, the owner should notify the insurance company before euthanasia is carried out. If there is even the slightest doubt as to whether the claim will be considered valid, the veterinarian concerned should obtain a second opinion from another experienced veterinarian. Insurance companies usually require a post mortem report with such a claim.

Cover for permanent loss of use costs much more than humane slaughter cover. Make sure which type of policy you require: all too often owners opt for the cheaper one, thinking that there is very little difference between them. There is a great deal of difference. A permanent loss of use policy pays out if the horse develops a problem which permanently prevents it from being used for a particular activity. Insurance companies usually group these activities into bands, with premiums reflecting the risk. So it costs more if the horse is going to be used for three day eventing than if it is just going to be used for hacking. The insurance is against being able to take part in the activity, not to maintain the same level of success.

The loss of use must be permament, not just temporary. Usually this means that there is no prospect of the horse returning to work within a year. It is also dependent on all possible treatments having been tried, without success. The better insurance companies have a veterinary advisor who liaises with the owner's veterinarian to make sure that everything possible has been done for the horse. If the owner refuses to try a recognised treatment for a particular problem, then the policy is void.

Most loss of use policies provide for a payment of less than 100% of the insured value if the horse is still capable of some activities or breeding. There is great variation in the percentage payable. There is also variation over what happens if the horse is accepted as having no use whatsoever. Some companies require the horse to be slaughtered for human consumption in order to provide maximum carcase value for themselves. Other companies do not require any carcase value, and may not require euthanasia.

Whatever policy is taken out, the owner should notify the company immediately if the horse has any illness. This applies even if the horse is expected to make a complete recovery. Failure to do this may invalidate the policy. It is also important to mention any illness when renewing a policy. Horse policies such as I have been describing are not continuous, but require a separate policy for each year. If owners do not notify the company of everything at renewal, they may encounter problems such as those already mentioned in respect of pre-existing conditions and exclusions.

Inevitably, this section has a rather negative character. I have tried to point out the pitfalls of insurance, because the straightforward claims bring their own reward. The choice of insurance company is all-important. Cheap premiums often reflect an unwillingness to pay out on claims. Ask friends about their experiences, and ask your veterinarian for any suggestions.

Basic hygiene and disease prevention

It is a mistake to regard hygiene only in relation to the stable environment and any visitors to it. The horse itself is the greatest threat to stable hygiene. There is no point in worrying about other horses bringing disease into the yard when the resident horse went to a show two days previously and came into contact with a respiratory virus there. Ideally, a horse should be isolated every time it comes back from a show. This is impractical, of course, but I do think that if a horse is stabled away from home then it should be isolated to some extent when it returns. This may mean turning it out for a minimum of three days, or stabling it with as little contact with others as is possible.

A horse's stable can be a safe environment because it enables the horse to build up immunity to any minor infections present. Putting a horse into another horse's stable for even a relatively short time can expose it to 'foreign' infections, especially if the stable is in a different yard. Disease can result even though the existing inmate is perfectly healthy.

If a horse can bring disease onto the premises then so can the vehicle which carries that horse. By law, commercial carriers must disinfect their vehicles after every trip; private owners should adopt a similar practice. No matter how inconvenient it might be, a vehicle should be disinfected if it has been used to carry a 'foreign' horse. It has been shown that respiratory infections flourish in the conditions found in a vehicle on the move. It is likely that the journeying to and from an event is as much responsible for the horse coughing afterwards as is the mixing with infected horses while there.

The stable yard is the next culprit. While cleanliness can be carried too far, a minimum requirement for the yard is that it be kept free from any urine drainage or faeces, because bacteria tend to multiply rapidly in such conditions *(Fig. 35)*. As a general rule, hay and straw should never be stored in the stable yard, but kept elsewhere, where the prevailing wind cannot blow fungal spores from them directly into the horse's lungs.

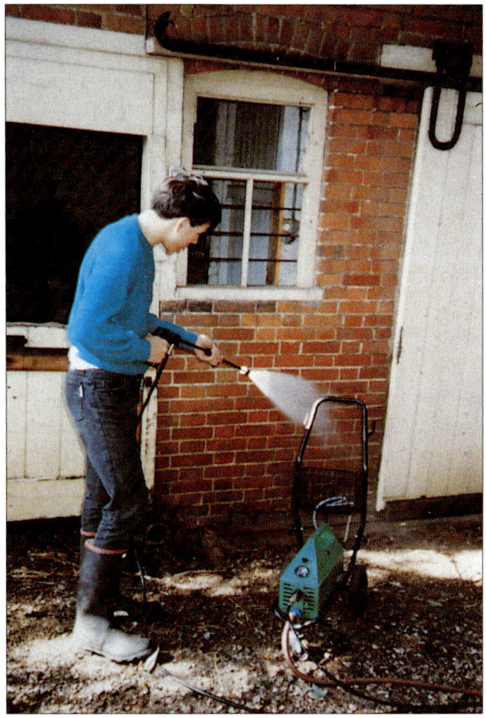

Fig. 35 *Hosing down stables*

Keeping horses in barns, where several stables and their access passageway are under one roof, can be very pleasant for the people looking after the horses in poor weather. Unfortunately it also ensures the rapid spread of any airborne infections. Often, too, conventional stables opening onto a yard have no partitions between stables in the roof spaces, and there is mixing of air along the line. A respiratory infection in one horse will thus spread rapidly to the others, and fungal spores from a stable bedded with straw will pass to a horse bedded on shavings.

Every stable should have a clean air inlet and an air outlet. This ideal is not achieved very often. In many stables the top stable door is the only air inlet. If this is the case then that door should never be

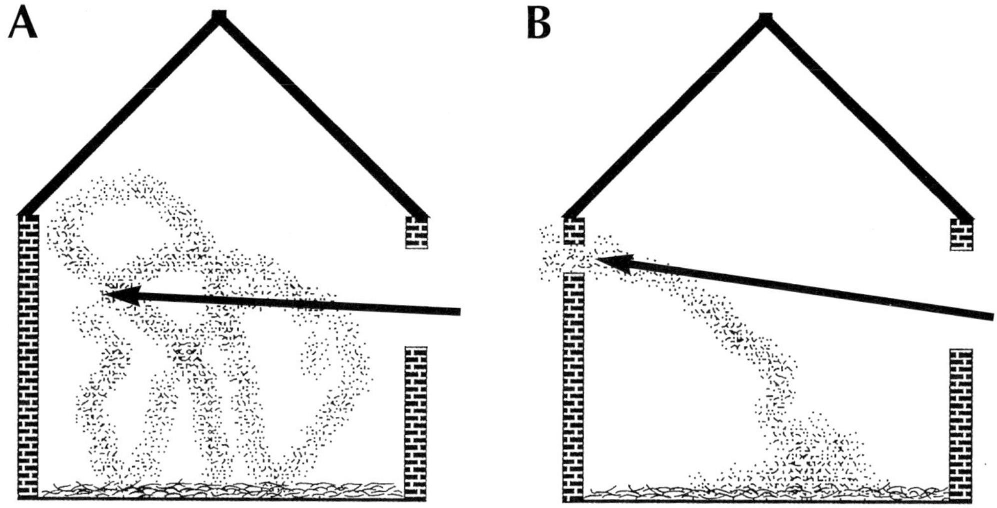

Fig. 36 *(A) With no through ventilation, dust and fungal spores from bedding are recirculated. (B) Ventilation through open top door or window removes dust and fungal spores from bedding.*

shut for more than an hour at a time. If we assume that an average horse weighs as much as seven people, and then imagine the atmosphere if seven people lived, slept, ate, urinated and defecated in a closed room the size of a stable, then the need for ventilation should be obvious. If the stable does not already have an air outlet, one should be installed either along the roof ridge or the eaves *(Fig. 36)*.

It is more important to keep the stable clean than to disinfect it regularly. Very few infections can survive for any length of time exposed to drying and sunlight, but, if protected by dust and dirt, they can survive for long periods. If a horse has an infectious disease, its stable should be disinfected every couple of days both to speed its recovery and to prevent disease spreading. Care should be taken to use a disinfectant which is active in the presence of organic material. Check that the instructions for the disinfectant state that it is active in such circumstances. A product that includes a detergent to aid the removal of organic material is the ideal choice.

Planning for health

Owners should not expect their horses to lead long and active lives without any planning. It is a good idea to obtain or draw up a week-by-week year planner. Mark down everything which affects a horse's health—things which need to be done and those which have been done. Our memories are fallible, and seeing everything spread out before us helps us to plan wisely.

An example of this is a horse's vaccination programme. Routine vaccinations are always best followed by rest rather than stress. This applies to both tetanus and equine influenza vaccinations. Paradoxically, the influenza vaccine will probably state this specifically in the written instructions, yet the tetanus vaccine is more likely to provoke a local reaction.

Owners tend to come back from holiday or get their horse up from grass full of enthusiasm, and it's then that they remember routine vaccinations. Immunity levels, however, are mostly higher, and the incidence of side effects lower, if vaccinations are given before the rest. Mark on the chart when the vaccination will need to be given—just before the 'holiday' preceding the date when the annual booster really must be given. If there is more than one horse in the yard, try to have them all done on the same day: a veterinary surgeon's visit costs more than the actual vaccination.

The diseases against which vaccination is possible vary from country to country. In the UK, vaccinations exist against equine influenza, tetanus, equine viral arteritis (EVA) or equine herpes virus 1 (EHV1), while in the United States protection is additionally available against equine herpes virus 4, Western, Eastern and Venezualan equine encephalitis, Potomac horse fever, rabies and strangles. It may or may not be appropriate to vaccinate against each disease at very different times during the year. Mares are usually best vaccinated one or two months before foaling, in order to ensure that they have maximum levels of antibodies present to pass via the colostrum to the foal.

You should next decide how frequently a horse is going to be shod, and, together with the farrier, mark those weeks on the planner. If the interval is longer than eight weeks, you will be riding a horse with improperly balanced feet. If for any reason a shoeing has to be delayed, do not put back the next date. If you do, you may find at the end of the year that the horse has been shod four or five times rather than six or seven. The difference might not seem much, but the extra stresses and strains on the feet may be significant.

The third step is to plan the deworming programme. Veterinarians are only too happy to help their clients with advice on special factors relating to their problems or locality. Deworming should normally be carried out every eight weeks. Whichever drug is used routinely, it is important to use one which is active against bots at the worming nearest to December, which is the period when the larvae are present in the stomach. It is also sensible to worm immediately before turning out to grass and immediately after a stabling period begins. If a horse has to go away while its owner is on holiday, then it should be wormed on its return with a drug which is effective against worm larvae.

Pregnant mares pose slightly different problems. The whole system will revolve around the expected foaling months. Note that I use the word 'months' rather than 'days'. A mare can give birth to a perfectly normal, full-term foal up to a month before or a month after the 340th day, which is considered the 'normal' foaling date. Ideally, therefore, we should complete our preparations around a month before we expect the mare to foal. If the mare is going away to stud to foal, she should do so well ahead of the expected date, so that she has a chance to build up good antibody levels against any infections present on the stud. A very simple test can tell you when a mare is getting close to foaling. This involves adding a few drops of 'milk' from the mare's udder to a solution, and looking at the colour change on a special paper strip. A positive reaction indicates that the mare will probably foal in the next twelve hours.

Many stallion owners require swabs to be taken from a mare before she visits the stallion, in order to ensure that she is not carrying infections such as contagious equine metritis (CEM) or other venereal diseases (see page 97). When a stallion is selected to mate a mare, check the swabbing requirements and enter them on the year planner so that they do not get forgotten. Later, pregnancy testing often needs to be carried out at precise times to confirm whether a further payment is necessary to the stallion owner. It is in the mare owner's interest to ensure that these requirements are met, otherwise he or she will be liable for the payment even if the mare is no longer pregnant.

Every horse should have its teeth checked at least once a year, and this should be entered on the planner. Horses being asked to perform very precise work such as dressage may benefit from more frequent checking. In my opinion it is not possible to rasp or float a horse's teeth without the use of a gag to hold the jaws properly apart. This enables the veterinarian to examine the teeth carefully before and after the rasping, and ensures that the rasps can be moved along the whole arcade of teeth. It is usual to use an angled head for rasping or floating the upper teeth and a straight head for the lower teeth. As a rule the outside edges of the upper teeth and the inside edges of the lower teeth need to be rasped.

I am impressed when walking into a tack room to see a blackboard detailing each horse's diet. Unfortunately, weeks or months later the same entries are often still on the board. Feeding schedules must be flexible, following the needs of both horse and trainer. When a significant change is made in the amounts that are fed—for example, if the quantity of an ingredient is altered by more than half a pound—then the new formula should be written on the planner. It is also worth noting why the formula has been changed. If the horse is losing weight when performing a certain amount of work, then recording that fact may save the owner making the same mistake again.

The final stage in preparing the master plan is to enter any background information available on each horse. As discussed earlier, its resting heart or pulse rate and resting respiratory rate should be known and entered there. If any 'healthy' blood samples have been taken, their levels can be entered for comparison with any 'disease' levels which might be taken later.

The discipline which is needed to keep a horse's health planned and recorded on paper can also be applied to planning a 'start-up' routine every time the horse is exercised. Before the horse is taken out of the stable, flex all four legs by holding them up and fully bent for several seconds. The front legs should also be extended forwards and straight (or rather, partially bent because the horse must bend the leg when it comes forward). Next, each leg should be examined, feeling for any unusual heat or swelling.

When the horse is brought out of the stable or field, it should be trotted away and back for 20–30 yards in hand. This will further loosen up the muscles of movement. It helps to have another person present, to observe the horse's locomotion from a different viewpoint; they should be able to tell whether the horse's head nods or its backside sinks down as it trots along. Once a rider climbs into the saddle, the opportunity to detect mild lameness is lost. The observer doesn't have to be an expert, nor need he or she know on which leg the horse is lame. It is sufficient to know that there is a problem, so that the necessary steps can be taken to deal with it. As discussed earlier, the horse nods when its good front leg takes the weight, and its hindquarters sink when its good hind leg takes the weight.

Second opinions and further investigations

I cannot stress too much the advantages of forming a good working relationship with a particular veterinary advisor. It will help to ensure that you obtain the kind of service which horse owners now have a right to expect. However, there will be times when a horse will not respond to treatment as well or as quickly as expected. Owners may then doubt whether their veterinary advisor has made the correct diagnosis or whether there are better treatments available.

If this happens, express those doubts to the veterinarian clearly but diplomatically. They may already feel that a rethink is necessary anyway. If the owner is still not satisfied (or if the veterinarian is not satisfied) then a second opinion should be obtained. It is important that you obtain the veterinarian 's permission to do so. Do not simply contact a veterinarian who appears most popular at that time. Veterinarians are not allowed to look at horses which have already been treated by somebody else unless they have that person's permission. If a second opinion is desirable, then ideally the original veterinarian should arrange it. This ensures that direct conflict between drugs and treatments is avoided.

A second opinion is only worthwhile if it adds something to the first, either by way of experience, or facilities, or both. If lameness is the problem, the horse should ideally go to someone with an interest in lameness rather than an expert on breeding problems. Even with large specialist equine practices and university departments there may be no advantage in seeking the advice of a recent graduate in preference to that of a local practitioner with many years' experience. It may be, therefore, that owners will have to travel a considerable distance to obtain a second opinion. It is worthwhile doing so if it means getting the best advice available.

If the second opinion differs from that of the original veterinarian, it should not be considered as reflecting badly on the previous advisor. In reaching a different opinion, the most crucial factor was probably the fact that the first treatment was unsuccessful. Hindsight is a great help on such occasions.

Occasionally owners may feel that a veterinary advisor who has acted for them has been negligent in treating or examining their horse or has acted unprofessionally. If that is the case, then it is only right that they should seek redress via the courts and consult a lawyer. Almost all veterinary advisors have insurance against such claims, and the insurance companies involved are very experienced in defending them. The success rate of negligence claims against veterinarians is generally very low, a statistic of which the profession has a right to be proud. In assessing whether anyone has been negligent, the crtieria are not whether the treatment was successful or the opinion was correct. The deciding factor is whether other veterinary surgeons would have done the same thing in the same circumstances. Again, all elements of hindsight have to be ignored.

If it is considered that a veterinarian has behaved unethically, a complaint should be addressed directly to the profession's ruling body (see appendix page 172). In the UK, a preliminary investigation committee will liaise between the complainant and the veterinarian concerned, and if its members think there may be a valid case, a disciplinary committee hearing will be called.

This committee has many of the powers of a court of law. Its ultimate sanction is the withdrawal of the veterinarian's right to practice. Such a hearing is concerned solely with apportioning blame and penalising anyone found guilty. It has no power to award damages to the complainant. That is a civil court matter. Contrary to some opinion, professional bodies such as the Royal College of Veterinary Surgeons do not act to protect the vets, or even the public. They are charged first and foremost with safeguarding the interests of the animals, who cannot speak for themselves.

There is a Guide to Professional Conduct which advises veterinarians on what is and what is not acceptable. This has changed over the years, mirroring changes in public opinion, but its underlying ethos has remained consistent—to assess whether an action could in some way be against an animal's best interests. In the U.S.A. each state has a board of Veterinary Medicine which licenses veterinarians to practise in that state. The board may withdraw that licence if a disciplinary hearing so decides. Many states automatically refuse to license veterinarians who have previously had their licence withdrawn elsewhere.

There should be few, if any, occasions when the relationship between owner and veterinarian breaks down. If it does, an owner wishing to transfer veterinary care to someone else should notify the veterinarian of their intention to contact another practice. It is inadvisable to change practices in mid-treatment if it can possibly be avoided. Before changing to a specialist equine practice some distance away, make sure that a local practice is prepared to provide emergency cover for wounds, acute colic and so on where travelling time might be important. Naturally the fee for such emergency treatment might reflect the fact that the owner is not also providing the more profitable routine work for the practice.

Euthanasia

One of the differences between human and veterinary medicine is that veterinarians are responsible for carrying out euthanasia, ensuring a rapid, painless death by artificial means. This is usually carried out either by the intravenous injection of a drug or by shooting with a pistol using special ammunition. From the horse's point of view I do not think there is much to choose between the two methods.

Shooting is more dramatic but is so instantaneous that the horse knows nothing about it. There is some risk to surrounding personnel, and the noise draws attention to the act, especially at crowded equine events. The injection of drugs involves an overdose of a drug which could in other circumstances be used to induce anaesthesia. Because of the volume of injection needed the horse has to stand reasonably still for several seconds while the procedure is being carried out. Then there is a short delay before the horse collapses to the ground. However, there is no question of the horse feeling any sensation other than that we feel when succumbing to a general anaesthetic. Whichever method is used, there may be some reflex muscle movements for a minute or so afterwards, including what may appear to be breathing movements. I should also point out that a dead animal will still have its eyes open – a fact which comes as quite a shock to some people.

With growing legislation on hygiene and environmental matters throughout the world, the disposal of the carcases of horses not slaughtered for meat can be quite a problem. Burial pits must be very deep and must avoid contamination of water courses. In the UK the traditional knackermen who collected animal carcases have all but disappeared, and in some countries they have gone completely. Hunt kennels still provide the service but legislation threatens this, as it does the hunt's continued existence. Cremation is a practical alternative, albeit an expensive one, and some animal crematoria can provide a service for horses.

4: Respiratory function and disease

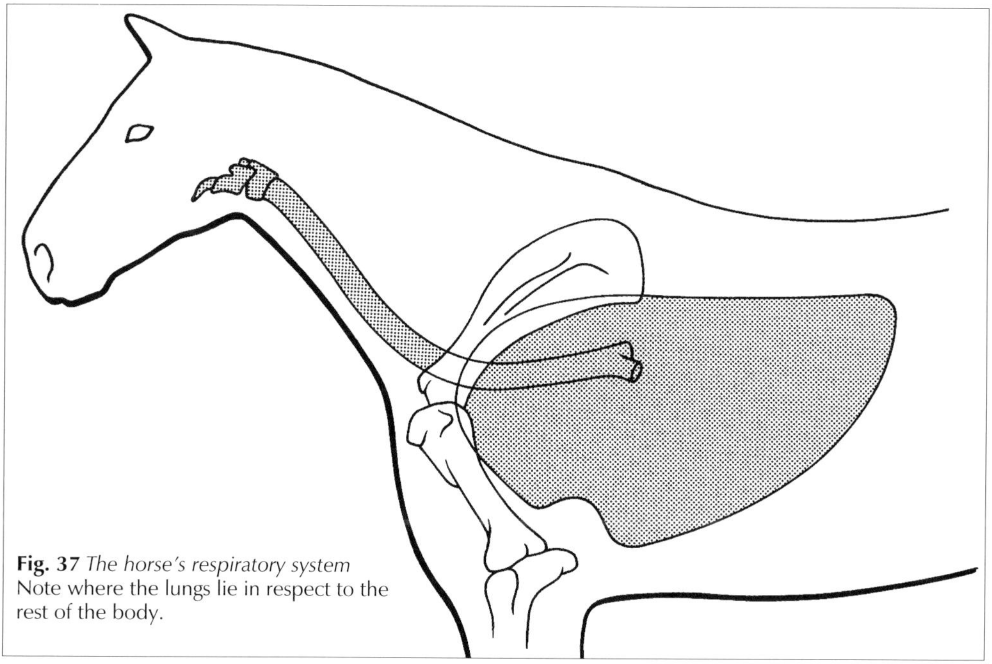

Fig. 37 *The horse's respiratory system*
Note where the lungs lie in respect to the rest of the body.

All parts of the horse's body need oxygen, which is obtained through the respiratory system *(Fig. 37)*. Air is drawn in from the nostrils to the lungs, five or more feet away in the thoracic, or chest, cavity. Here the air comes into close contact with the blood (although there is always at least one cell thickness between the two media). There is no active mechanism to ensure that the blood absorbs oxygen from the air; it is purely a passive movement. The oxygen is drawn from the air, where it is in a high concentration, to the blood simply because there is a much lower concentration of oxygen in the blood. At the same time, carbon dioxide, which is in a high concentration in the blood coming into the lungs, will pass in the opposite direction into the air. The rate of gas exchange cannot be increased, even if the body needs extra oxygen.

Air enters the body via the nostrils. These are very mobile in the horse. They can be dramatically dilated to ensure as large an air intake as possible when the horse is frightened (and wants to run away) or exhausted from exercise. Note that, for reasons which will be explained later, the horse breathes through its nostrils and cannot breathe through its mouth. Inside the nose, air passes over the turbinate bones. These are rather complicated bones which are scroll-shaped in cross-section so that they pre-

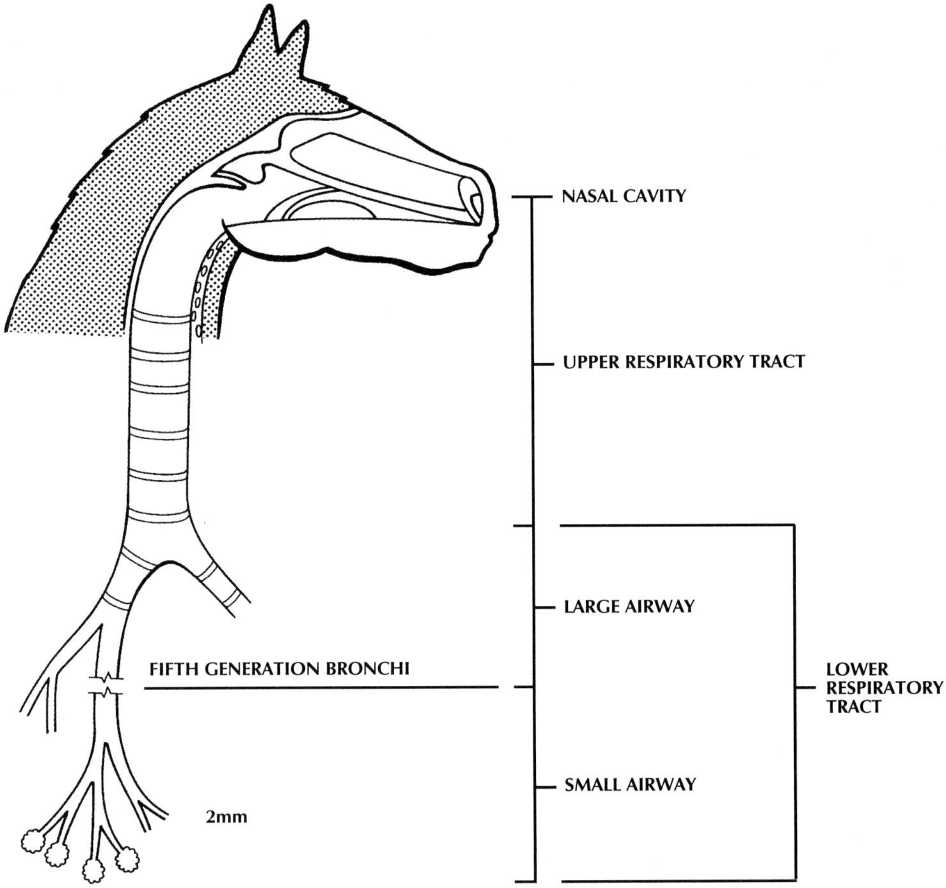

Fig. 38 *The respiratory system*
Note how the diameter of the tubes gets smaller and smaller until they end in an alveolus.

sent as large a surface area to the air as possible. The surface is covered with a plexus of small blood vessels which act rather like the elements of an electric fan heater. As the air passes over the blood vessels of the turbinates it warms up. This prevents freezing cold air coming into contact with the sensitive lung tissue. If horses are being trained at fast speeds in very low or sub-zero temperatures, they may need to be fitted with a special hood which creates turbulence (and so warming) of the air even before it enters the nostrils. In such conditions the warming effect of the turbinates alone is insufficient *(Fig. 38)*.

The air then enters the pharynx, a cavity at the back of the mouth. In man the pharynx contains two distinct structures, the tonsils, whose function is to trap infectious agents before they get further down the respiratory tract. The horse does not have tonsils. It does, however, have lymphoid tissue which deals with infection in a similar way. This is dispersed over the roof of the pharynx.

If an infection is present, droplets of purulent mucus hang from the roof of the pharynx. This can be seen using an instrument called a fibreoptic endoscope, a long flexible tube with two bundles of very fine glass fibres running the length of the endoscope *(Fig. 39)*. A bright light source is beamed down one set of fibres to illumi-

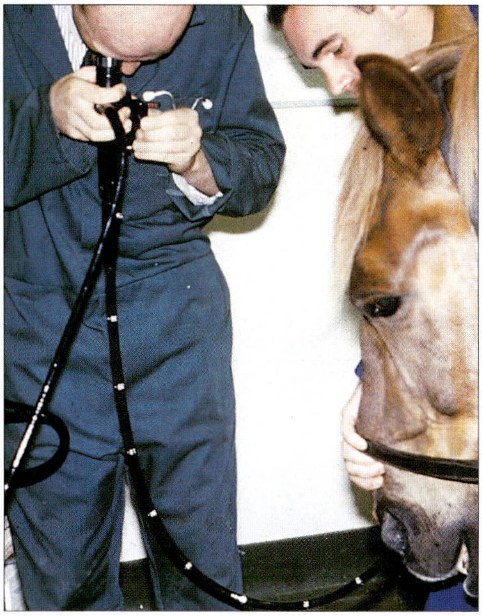

Fig. 39 *An endoscopic examination*

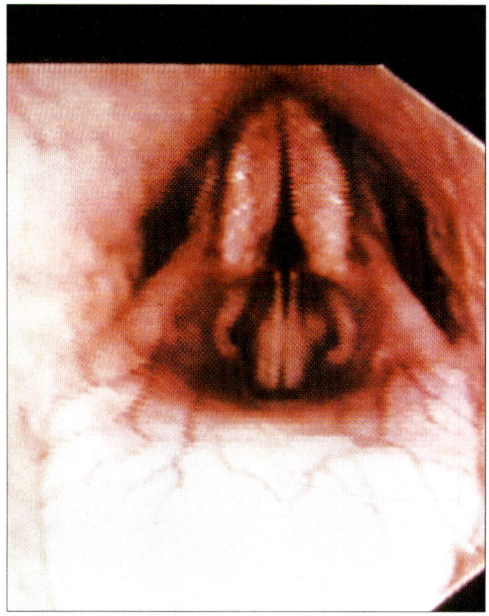

Fig. 40 An endoscopic view of a normal horse's larynx.

nate the area around the tip. Through the eyepiece it is possible to see, via the second fibre bundle, the view from the tip of the endoscope *(Fig. 40)*.

Entering into each side of the pharynx are the eustachian tubes which link the pharynx with the middle ear, equalising the atmospheric pressure. If you have ever swallowed hard to relieve painful pressure in your ears as an aeroplane lands you have been been using your eustachian tubes. In man they are straightforward tubes, but in the horse they balloon out to form guttural pouches in the region directly below each ear.

As I mentioned earlier, the horse cannot breathe through its mouth. This is because for most of the time the larynx (voice box), and trachea (windpipe), are cut off from the mouth cavity by the soft palate. This is a sheet of membrane which is the continuation of the roof of the mouth (the hard palate). The horse's larynx protrudes through a hole in this soft palate. This ensures that food particles from the mouth cannot get into the trachea and lungs. When the horse wants to swallow some food, it has to stop breathing and pull the larynx out of the soft palate while closing the entrance to the larynx. The food bolus then goes into the oesophagus (see page 65, Digestive System) and the larynx returns to its resting position.

The larynx is a rigid structure consisting of both muscle and cartilage. It is basically a cylinder which is open at both ends. At the rear it fits directly into the trachea. At the front there are two arytenoid cartilages which can either be held together across the entrance or pulled upwards and to the side. Attached to these cartilages are folds of membrane which form the vocal cords. As everyone knows the sounds any animal makes when communicating are usually produced by controlling the air flow out over the vocal cords, and controlling the position of the vocal cords in that airflow. At rest the arytenoid cartilages are held only slightly open, but when the horse starts to exercise they are gradually pulled open to allow more air into the trachea.

The trachea is simply a tube extending

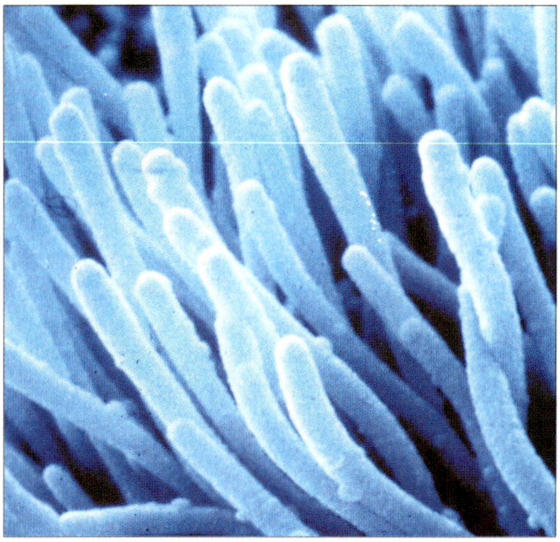

Fig. 41 An electron microscope view of the cilia lining a horse's trachea.

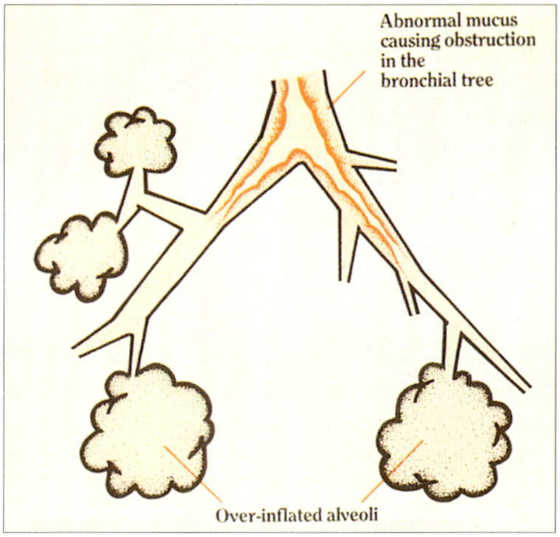

Fig. 42 The effects of mucus blocking the horse's airway.

down to the lungs. Its lining appears to be smooth, but in fact it is covered with millions of fine hairs called cilia *(Fig. 41)*. These move in waves from the bottom of the trachea upwards towards the larynx. They provide a kind of escalator which carries mucus up from the lungs to the mouth where it will either be swallowed or coughed out. Some horses are very effective 'swallowers' of mucus and so cough very little. Others swallow hardly any of the mucus, and so cough much more frequently. The frequency of coughing is therefore not a reliable guide to the amount of mucus being produced. Unfortunately, virus infections can both slow the rate at which the cilia move and erode the hairs away, causing them to lose much of their ability to remove mucus just when they are needed most.

Before the airway reaches the lungs it divides into two. As it enters each lung, the airway subdivides into tubes which become progressively smaller. They begin as relatively large tubes called bronchi, which branch and branch again, getting smaller all the time. The smallest tubes are called bronchioles. As mentioned above, the trachea is rigid, because its airway is protected by rings of cartilage. At the other end of the system the bronchioles have only thin walls, without any cartilage, and their diameter can be altered by the contraction or relaxation of muscles in the bronchiolar wall.

The purpose of the lungs is to provide a large area for gas exchange between the air and the bloodstream. This takes place in a great number of tiny sacs called alveoli. Think of the alveoli as the leaves of the tree: they are the active powerhouse of the system. The branching bronchioles and bronchi are the branches and the trachea is the equivalent of the trunk through which all the sap flows. The alveolar walls are basically only one cell thick, with the network of tiny blood vessels running between the walls of the adjacent alveoli. The efficiency of the system is helped by the fact that the surfaces in contact with the air are covered with thin mucus which is constantly replaced. Oxygen dissolves readily in this mucus and then travels across the cell barrier. The resting horse only fully utilises a proportion of the available alveoli.

When a horse enters a dusty atmosphere, it is natural to think that dust will penetrate right down into the lungs. In fact this doesn't happen. The heavier particles fall to the floor of the large airways within a relatively short distance. The lighter the dust particle, the further it penetrates into the small airways. Therefore, the dust we see in the stable is not really a problem; the real danger to the lungs comes from the fine dust particles which we cannot see. These include physical irritants such as virus particles and fungal spores.

A cough tends to be regarded as undesirable. Owners may put up with a horse breathing heavily, but want instant treatment to put an end to any coughing which develops. In fact, we should encourage any coughing that develops because it is a protective mechanism. When a horse coughs there is a violent expulsion of air from the lungs. This picks up and carries with it a great deal of the mucus *(Fig. 42)* and dust particles over which that air travels. We distinguish between a dry cough or a moist, productive cough. While a moist cough means that there is considerable mucus present in the airway, a dry cough does not necessarily denote an absence of mucus. The mucus may have become thick and tacky, or tenacious, so that even though the horse coughs it fails to move or dislodge it. As a result the horse coughs even more frequently, each time attempting to move the same globule of mucus.

As the horse continues coughing there is an increased risk of the physical act of coughing causing a sore throat. A vicious circle can then develop where the horse coughs because of the throat irritation but has the irritation because of the cough *(Fig. 43)*. One of the reasons why horses sometimes cough when they start exercise is that the sudden influx of cooler air taken in at that time irritates the inflamed membranes and triggers a cough. Another

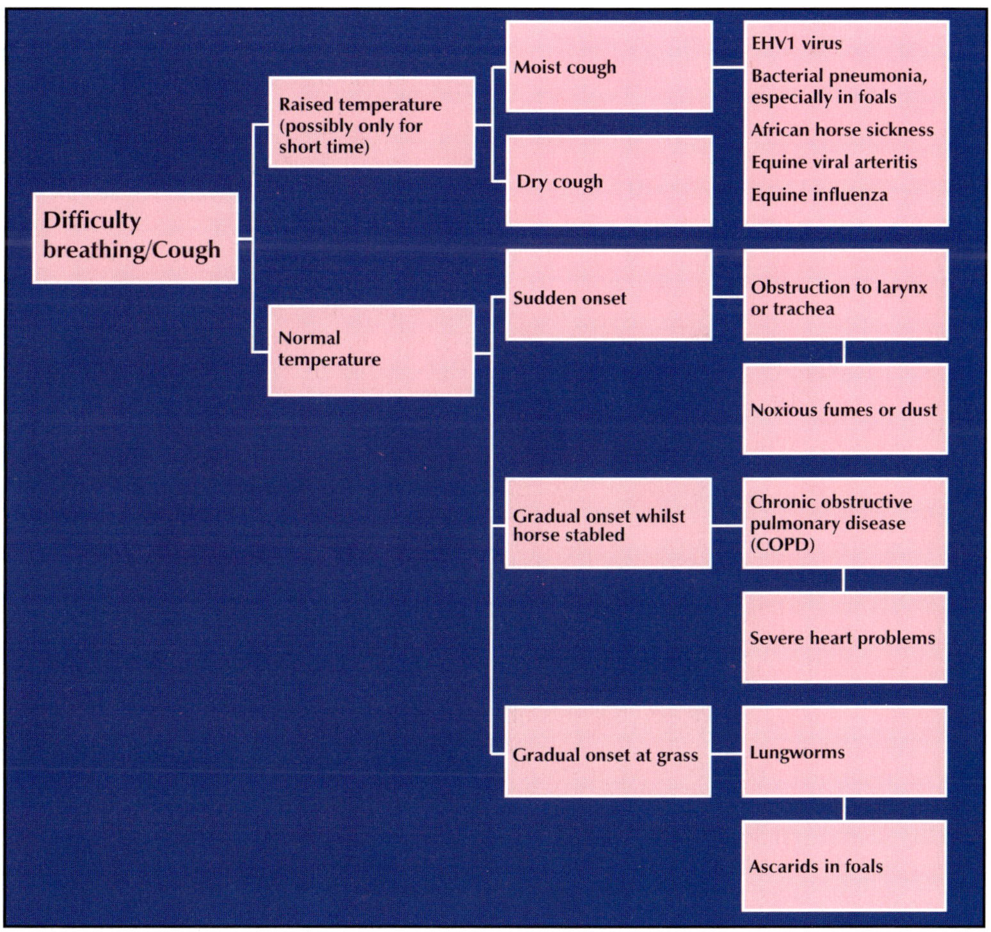

Fig. 43 *The coughing horse*

reason is that the excitement of exercise causes the release of adrenaline into the horse's bloodstream. Adrenaline causes bronchodilation, or opening of the small airways. As a result mucus can more readily escape and be coughed out.

The opposite of bronchodilation is broncho-constriction. This occurs when the muscles of the bronchiolar walls contract and reduce the diameter of the airway. Physical irritants such as fungal spores, dust particles and to a lesser extent virus particles can stimulate the bronchiolar lining and cause a reflex broncho-constriction. An allergic inflammatory reaction can have the same, but more lasting, effect. Broncho-constriction reduces airflow through the airway, and can also prevent the removal of thick mucus.

Because so many horses are kept as athletic animals, it is worth giving more detailed information on how the horse's respiratory tract responds to increased oxygen demand during and after exercise. The nostrils can be opened more widely, so that the cross-sectional area of the aperture increases to match the cross-section of the passageways up the nose and over the turbinates. This is more important than some people might imagine. It is true that we very rarely have problems which prevent the horse opening its nostrils as required, but that does not alter the fact that the airflow is limited by its narrowest point, whether that occurs at the nostrils, or further along, for example in the larynx.

The next adaptation occurs in the larynx. At rest the two arytenoid cartilages almost meet in the centre of the laryngeal airway. As more and more air is needed by the lungs, the cartilages are held more and more open, increasing the airway. It is possible to overestimate the importance of minor variations in the movement of these cartilages. They affect the airflow but may not limit performance because there may still be sufficient air available. Owners should appreciate that the airway from the nostrils to the lungs is otherwise of a fixed diameter, and cannot increase airflow for exercise.

There is also a so-called 'dead space' of air in the system. The first air a horse breathes in is the air already in the upper airway. This is, however, the last air to be expelled from the lungs during the previous breath, high in carbon dioxide and low in oxygen.

The lungs adapt to the needs of exercise in several ways. First, the adrenaline released causes bronchodilation, increasing the amount of air which can pass through the bronchioles. Second, the number of bronchioles and alveoli which are used can be increased. Ideally, a galloping horse will be fully expanding all its alveoli, although disease may limit this.

Thirdly the horse can increase the number of breaths it takes in any fixed time. We all know that a horse will be breathing more quickly after exercise, and this will continue for some time until the horse has 'repaid' all the oxygen needed to produce the energy used up during exercise. What is less well-known is that at the canter and the gallop the respiratory rate is linked to the stride rate—so a horse cannot take more breaths per minute than it takes strides. If a horse has some problem which limits the amount of air reaching the alveoli during the gallop, it cannot, therefore, compensate by breathing any more rapidly, because the muscles which expand the chest are also those which help to pull the forelegs forward. There is no such fixed link between stride and emptying the lungs because this is a passive operation. Any disease which decreases the efficiency of lung emptying allows less room in the lungs for oxygen-rich air to be sucked in at the next breath. Finally exercise increases the heart rate, and so increases the blood supply to the lungs. This enables more oxegen to be picked up if it is available.

Disease prevention

The prevention of respiratory problems depends on the avoidance of respiratory infections and the provision of clean air at all times. Respiratory infections are usually spread in the air, carried by tiny droplets of mucus which have been coughed up, or by dust particles. There does not need to be direct physical contact between a healthy horse and an infected one to pass the infection on. Virus particles, for instance, can be carried by the wind for hundreds of metres. This makes isolation of an infected horse very difficult. Even if we move the horse far away from its stable companions, infective particles will still be blowing on the wind. So, for practical purposes there is no point in trying to isolate a horse once it has developed a respiratory infection. We will almost certainly be too late.

The aim must therefore be to prevent the introduction of such infections into the yard in the first place. Vaccines have a role to play in protecting against some respiratory infections. However, with most of the vaccines presently available it takes five to six weeks from the time of the first vaccination to the time of maximum protection. They do not therefore have a role to play in preventing the spread of existing disease within a stable yard—the incubation period of such infections is only around three to ten days. Two other important factors affect the efficacy of vaccines. One is that at least 80% of the horses at risk need to have been vaccinated if vaccines are to provide maximum protection, so we have to persuade all the owners using the yard to vaccinate their horses. Secondly, vaccines are more effective when a number of doses have been given over a period. A horse that has had a number of doses of equine influenza vaccine over the years will be able to withstand a higher challenge than a horse that has only recently completed its initial vaccine course.

Whatever the cause of the inflammation in the respiratory system, the presence of any fine particles of matter in the atmosphere will cause irritation and so prolong the problem *(Fig. 44)*. In this respect, virus particles, hair particles from clipping, bacteria, hay and straw fragments and fungal spores are all undesirable. A horse with any inflammation is best taken off straw, which is likely to contain fungal spores, and put on wood shavings, peat or shredded paper. Even these alternative beddings can pose a danger if a deep litter system is used. The best bedding when treating respiratory problems is grass—that is, no stabling at all. Hay is also a threat, so Horseage or a complete high fibre ration such as hay cubes or alfalfa pellets should be fed *(Fig. 45)*. Damping hay has little effect in preventing fungal spores from being released over the number of hours most horses take to consume a hay net. If the horse has to be stabled, make sure that it is not

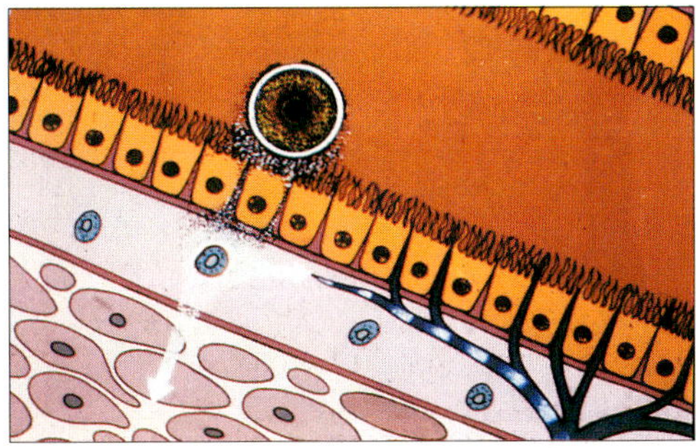

Fig. 44 A microscopic view of a pollen grain in contact with the lining of the bronchiole.

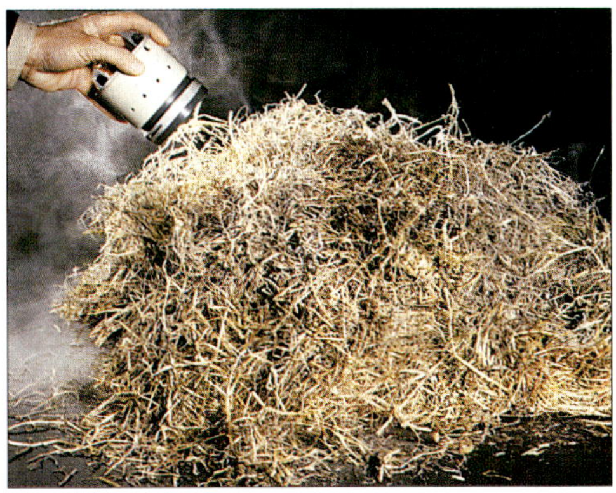

Fig. 45 Sampling the dust given off by hay using a slit sampler which sucks air in and deposits any particles on a specially prepared microscopic slide.

Viruses which affect the horse's respiratory system		
Adenovirus	Affects foals	No vaccine
Equine Herpes Virus Type 1	Common everywhere Can also cause abortion	Vaccines available
Type 2	No clinical symptons	No vaccine
Type 3	Usually causes coital exanthema rather than respiratory symptoms	No vaccine
Type 4	Can also cause ataxia and paralysis	Vaccine available
Equine influenza Miami, Prague, Kentucky and Suffolk strains	Epidemics common when new strain arises	Vaccination should include strain responsible Some cross-immunity
Equine rhinovirus	Spread by biting midges Respiratory symptoms in acute forms	Vaccine needs to include specific strain
Equine viral arteritis	Spread by air droplets and by venereal route	Vaccination posible

Fig. 46 *The common respiratory viruses*

downwind of any straw or hay stacks. Also, shut off any gaps which might allow dusty air from adjacent stables to come through. Concentrate on through ventilation from the front to the back wall of the stable and then out. Avoid storing hay or straw in the same building as horses.

The rapid spread of respiratory infections, especially equine influenza, in unprotected populations of horses can lead to serious epidemics. Voluntary movement controls and cancellation of organised equine activities may then have a role to play in controlling the disease.

Adenovirus

Symptoms Usually only foals are affected. They may develop a cough and a nasal discharge. Pneumonia may cause breathing difficulties. The foal may have a fever.

Cause An adenovirus infects the whole body, although it is the respiratory system which displays symptoms *(Fig. 46)*.

Treatment There are no antiviral drugs or vaccines available.

Prognosis Arabians seem particularly susceptible. Immunodeficient arabian foals will almost certainly be killed by the virus, but other breeds may show few or no symptoms.

Atheroma

Symptoms A swelling in the tissue under the skin of the false nostril. It is usually only of cosmetic importance.

Cause A tumour of skin tissue.

Treatment Surgical removal is fairly easy.

Prognosis Good after removal.

Chronic obstructive pulmonary disease (COPD)

Symptoms Mostly affects housed horses. The horse has a chronic cough and a nasal discharge. Even at rest its respiratory rate may be over 20 per minute. It has difficulty in emptying its lungs and has to consciously squeeze air out, giving a two part exhalation ('broken' wind) *(Fig. 47)*. Enlargement of the muscles involved may result in a 'heave line' along the side of the abdomen. Affected horses have a reduced ability to work. Permanent breakdown of the tiny air pockets in the lung (emphysema) is rare.

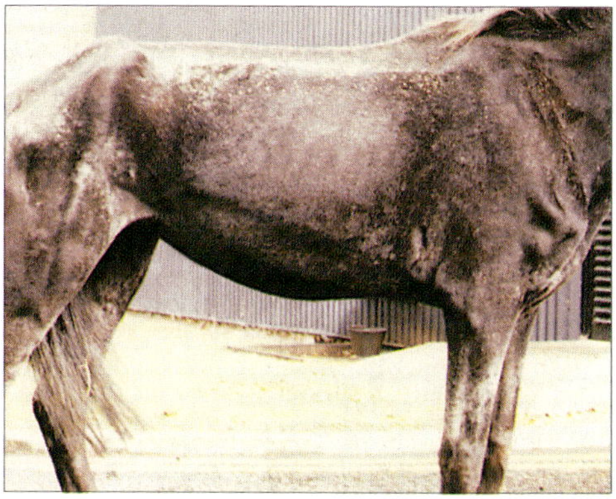

Fig. 47 *A horse with COPD*
Note the sloping heave line running forward across the abdomen from the stifle region.

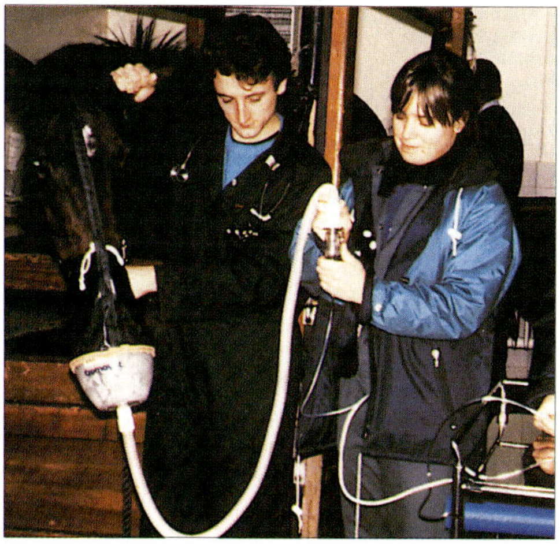

Fig. 48 Treating a horse with COPD using a nebuliser to enable it to breathe in a fine mist of drug particles.

Cause The breathing difficulties result from a constriction of the tiny airways, or bronchioles, in the lung. This is triggered by an allergy to fine dust particles, usually fungal spores from hay and straw although pollen (especially oil seed rape) may also be involved. Mucus is formed by the irritated membranes, and this can be seen travelling up the trachea during an endoscopic examination.

Treatment Symptoms usually disappear when the horse is removed from the dust which triggers the condition. Spending time out at grass is ideal. If stabled, it should not have access to straw or hay, or air which has passed over them in other stables. Bronchodilators, such as clenbuterol, will reverse the broncho-constriction. Sodium cromoglycate may temporarily prevent the allergic reaction, and is given via a nebuliser *(Fig. 48)*.

Prognosis When a horse has an allergy, it is usually permanent. So permanent 'clean air' therapy will be needed. With attention to detail over stable management most horses can become symptom-free in time. Without treatment, the symptoms steadily increase as more and more airways close down.

Cleft palate
Symptoms A problem of young horses. Milk or food is seen draining out of the nostrils. Examination of the hard palate along the roof of the mouth shows a gap in the middle through which the food passes. Pneumonia may occur if the food material is sucked into the lungs.

Cause The problem is congenital.

Treatment Surgery has been tried to seal the cleft, but the success rate is not good.

Prognosis Poor. Affected animals are usually euthanased.

Epiglottal entrapment
Symptoms The horse makes an abnormal respiratory noise on exercise. It may cough and choke.

Cause Inflammation and swelling of the fold of membrane which links the epiglottis with the rest of the larynx. This pulls the epitglottis out of its normal position.

Treatment Surgery can be successful.

Prognosis Some affected horses do not appear to be inconvenienced at all.

Equine influenza

Symptoms Affected horses usually have a dry cough. They have a temperature of around 103°F (39.4°C). There is a nasal discharge which at first is clear and watery, but which tends to become thick and purulent. Even after a horse appears to have recovered, secondary problems may arise, such as damaged heart muscles and chronic inflammatory changes in the lung leading to chronic obstructive pulmonary disease, or bleeding from the nose after exercise. Equine influenza is a very contagious disease, which spreads rapidly from one horse to another.

Cause Influenza is caused by the equine influenza virus, of which there are two main strains. The type 1 virus was first isolated in Prague in 1956, and the type 2 virus in Miami in 1963. The strains are often referred to by the names of their place of origin. Some further variation occurs in the virus strains, but not to the extent which it does in human influenza. At present the Suffolk 89 strain is most commonly involved, a type 2 virus.

Treatment Although there are no drugs which will kill the virus, it is now recognised that it is important to treat the changes which occur in the lung. Bronchodilators such as clenbuterol and mucolytics may prevent the changes which lead to later secondary problems. Rest is also *essential,* and should be for *at least six weeks* after an active infection. Effective vaccines are available that protect against both type 1 and type 2 equine influenza. Ideally the vaccine should include components of the virus strains involved in the outbreak or currently causing clinical disease in the area.

Prognosis All susceptible (non-vaccinated) horses on the premises usually become affected. Equine influenza can cause death in foals.

Equine rhinovirus

Symptoms Affected horses may have a raised temperature for a few days. The lymph glands around the throat may be enlarged, there may be a nasal discharge.

Cause A virus.

Treatment No specific treatment exists, nor is any usually necessary. There are no vaccines available.

Prognosis The symptoms are usually mild, although the disease can be a problem where young horses are gathered together.

Ethmoid haematomata

Symptoms Often the first symptom is a severe haemorrhage from the nose, which may or may not be associated with exercise. Affected horses may also have a persistent bloody discharge from one nostril.

Cause A form of tumour of the blood vessels associated with the ethmoid bone at the back of the nose.

Treatment Surgical removal of the mass is the only form of treatment.

Prognosis Prognosis must be guarded as at any time a massive fatal haemorrhage may occur unless all the mass is removed.

Exercise induced pulmonary haemorrhage (EIPH)

Symptoms The visible symptom is bleeding from the nose after exercise, although the blood originates from the lungs, rather than the nose *(Fig. 49)*. The majority of racehorses have some haemorrhage in their lungs after strenuous exercise, but only in a small percentage is this severe enough to show externally. There is no direct correlation between the severity of the lung haemorrhage and the appearance of blood at the nostrils.

Cause Pathological changes in the top part of the lungs are triggered off by respiratory virus infections. There is an increase in the number of small blood vessels in this region, and it is these new vessels which rupture.

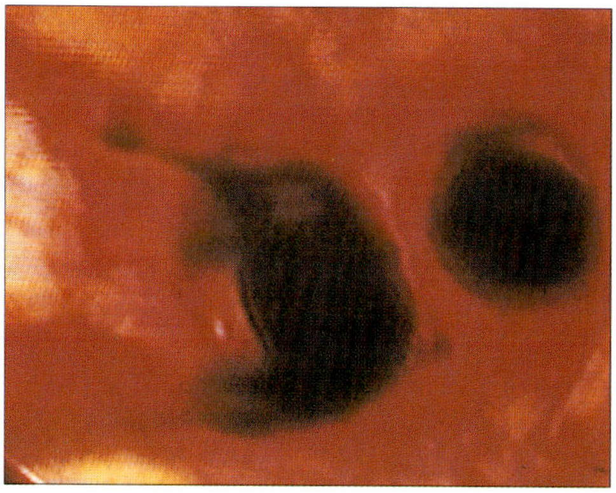

Fig. 49 *Endoscopic view of a horse's trachea*
Note the red blood coming up from the right lung (apparently on the left here because the camera is facing the horse).

Treatment The only treatment is to use bronchodilators and mucolytics to try to keep the airways open, especially during the initial infection. Frusemide has been used extensively in treatment. It has been shown to exert some bronchodilatory effect.

Prognosis The pathological changes are permanent and progressive. Any effect on performance is usually intermittent, particularly in the early stages of pathological change.

Foal pneumonia
Symptoms Foals have a raised temperature and obvious difficulty breathing. They may have a cough and/or a purulent nasal discharge. On X-ray abscesses may be visible in the lungs.

Cause The most serious organism involved is *Rhodococcus equi* (formerly known as *Corynebacterium equi*).

Treatment R. equi is very resistant to treatment with most antibiotics. Rifampin and erythrocin are the drugs of choice.

Prognosis Guarded, as *R. equi* abscesses can cause chronic problems and death in foals. Horses over six months old appear to be immune to the organism.

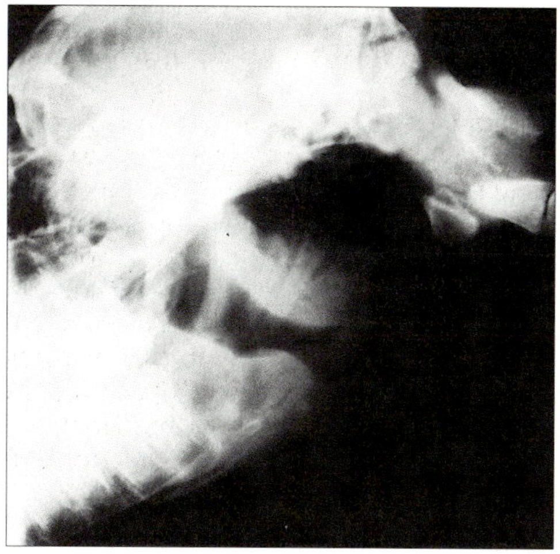

Fig. 50 *X-ray of a horse's skull*
The white mass in the upper left corner is a dense accumulation of pus in the guttural pouch.

Guttural pouch empyema
Symptoms A swelling appears in the area below the ear. This may obstruct the horse's airway and may even interfere with swallowing. The horse has a chronic, foul smelling nasal discharge. X-rays may show the pus/air boundary in the guttural pouch *(Fig. 50)*.

Cause Pus in the guttural pouch is usually secondary to infection and inflammation in the surrounding tissues (e.g. lymph nodes).

Treatment Drainage and flushing may be possible via a catheter through the pharyngeal opening. If the pus is dry and inspissated (has become thick), surgical removal will be needed.

Prognosis: Guarded.

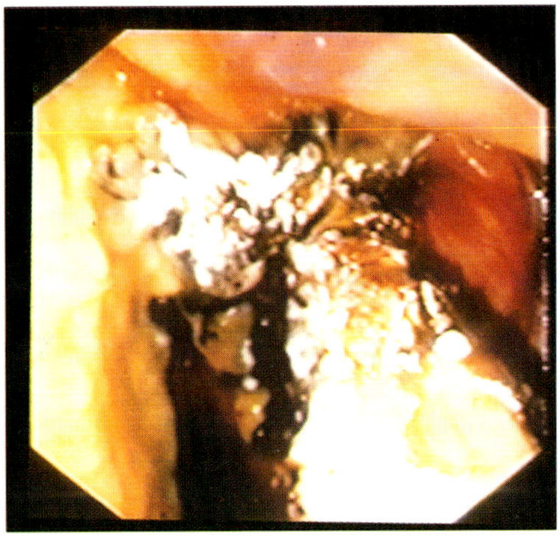

Fig. 51 *Endoscopic view of a horse's guttural pouch* The fungal growths are clearly visible.

Guttural pouch mycosis

Symptoms Bleeding from the nose may result in the loss of several litres of blood. The haemorrhage is not associated with exercise. An endoscopic examination shows that the blood is coming from one of the guttural pouches, which open off the pharynx. The roof of the pouch may be roughened *(Fig. 51)*.

Cause A fungal infection of the lining of the pouch, usually by Aspergillus. The fungus can involve the internal carotid artery. This results in stretching, and possibly rupture of the blood vessel immediately behind the constriction.

Treatment Antifungal drugs, administered in a variety of ways, have been used. Fresh air is very effective in killing the fungus and a catheter can be inserted between the pouch and a nostril to help in this way. If an artery is affected, and this can be ascertained using a special X-ray technique after a dye has been injected into the bloodstream, surgery is necessary to tie off the blood vessel to stop it rupturing again.

Prognosis Guarded.

Guttural pouch tympani

Symptoms A disease of young foals, especially fillies. A swelling develops below the ear which may cause respiratory distress or difficulty in swallowing. The swelling is drum-like when tapped with a finger.

Cause Usually a congenital problem with the pharyngeal opening.

Treatment An indwelling catheter allows passage of air into and out of the guttural pouch. Surgical relief may be necessary.

Prognosis Guarded.

Inhalation pneumonia

Symptoms Although pneumonia is relatively uncommon in adult horses, it can occur, with marked difficulty in breathing and an increased respiratory rate.

Cause Inhalation pneumonia can be caused by water entering the respiratory system during swimming. The commonest cause is fluid entering the respiratory system rather than the digestive system when owners attempt to treat horses by 'drenching' them (pouring medicine into the back of the mouth).

Treatment Antibiotics will control or prevent secondary infections while, hopefully, the original liquid is dealt with by the lung tissues.

Prognosis Guarded, depending on the liquid involved and the degree of secondary infection.

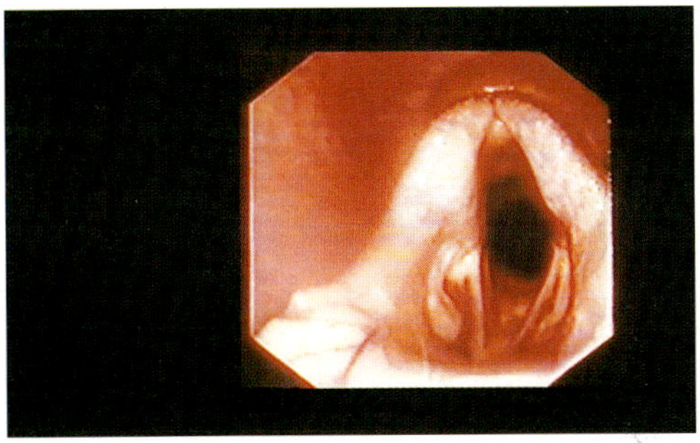

Fig. 52 *Endoscopic view of the larynx of a horse with left laryngeal hemiplegia.*
Note that the left side is less concave than the right as a result. The vet is standing facing the horse during the examination.

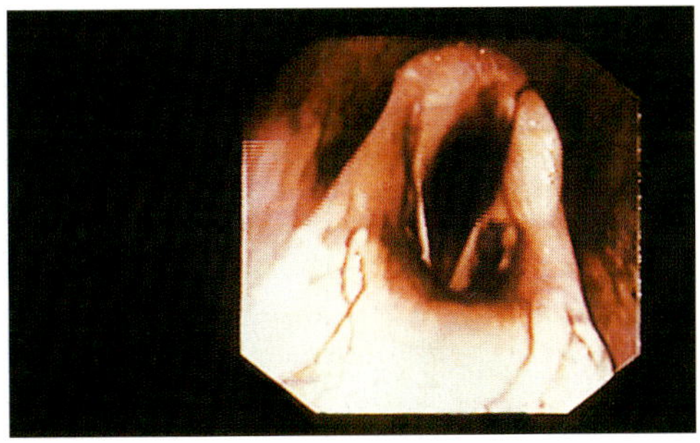

Fig. 53 *Endoscopic view of a horse's larynx after tieback surgery*
Note that the left side is now more concave than the right because it is fixed in the open position as if during exercise.

Laryngeal hemiplegia
Symptoms The horse makes a characteristic roaring noise when it breathes in during fast exercise. It may tire more readily than expected.

Cause A partial or complete paralysis of the muscles controlling the left vocal cord in the horse's larynx. The horse cannot pull the cartilage and fold of membrane out of the way to increase the size of the airway when it needs more oxygen. The paralysis is usually the result of an abnormality of the left recurrent laryngeal nerve, and the problem is usually present to some extent from birth *(Fig. 52)*. In some lines of horses it is an hereditary condition. Physical damage to the neck and acute viral damage to the nerve can occasionally also bring on the problem in previously symptom-free horses.

Treatment Treatment is only necessary if the problem affects the horse's ability to perform. The Hobday operation *may* reduce the noise by preventing air vibrating in the cavity behind the vocal cord (after its lining is stripped away during the operation scar tissue fills up the cavity). In the majority of horses, however, the operation fails to increase the size of the airway. The laryngeal prosthesis operation ties back the cartilage, so that the vocal cord is permanently in the position it occupies during fast exercise. This increases the diameter of the airway *(Fig. 53)*.

Prognosis Once the paralysis shows by causing the roaring noise, it will always do so. However other conditions, such as pharyngeal lymphoid hyperplasia (see page 50), can cause a similar noise and so the problem should always be evaluated by an endoscopic examination before considering surgery.

Lungworm
Symptoms Coughing develops in a horse which is out at grass. Often there is evidence that a donkey has been grazing the same pasture. There may be a nasal discharge. If the condition is allowed to persist, the horse may show symptoms similar to chronic obstructive pulmonary disease (COPD) (see page 44) as the small airways contract down.

Cause The lungworm is a parasite called *Dictyocaulus arnfieldi.* It is a common parasite in donkeys, where it causes few if any symptoms. In horses the worm larvae usually fail to mature and remain in the lungs as a chronic irritant. Symptoms usually start during the third week after the horse picks up the eggs on the pasture.

Treatment It is often difficult to arrive at a definite diagnosis of lungworm infestation because the larvae do not mature to egg-laying adults, and so faecal egg counts are not satisfactory. Treatment may be carried out in order to 'diagnose' the problem by removing any lungworms present. Ivermectin is effective against lungworm, as is a 10-times normal dose of thiabendazole (although this needs to be given via a stomach tube). Routine worming with other anthelmintics does not kill the parasite.

Prognosis Once a pasture has been contaminated with lungworms, it will reinfest horses every summer for a considerable number of years. If the lungs are permanently damaged, the horse may become hypersensitive to dust from hay and straw.

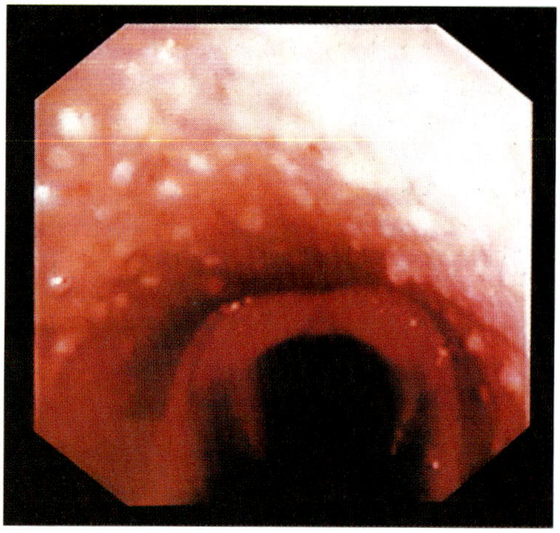

Fig. 54 *Endoscopic view of a horse's pharynx* The droplets of pus on the roof of the pharynx are associated with lymphoid hyperplasia.

Nasal polyps

Symptoms An abnormal noise during breathing, especially during strenuous exercise. Performance is not usually affected.

Cause One or more benign polyps growing from the wall of the nasal cavity just inside the nostrils.

Treatment If necessary surgical removal is possible.

Prognosis Rarely regrow after removal.

Pharyngeal lymphoid hyperplasia

Symptoms This is the equine version of tonsilitis. There are areas of lymphoid, or tonsillar, tissue scattered over the roof of the pharynx. When these are inflamed and infected, they can be seen during an endoscopic examination *(Fig. 54)*. Horses with this condition usually show no symptoms at all. On the other hand they usually make an abnormal respiratory noise, especially during fast work, and perform poorly.

Cause The lymphoid tissue is reacting to a variety of respiratory infections as part of the horse's immune response.

Treatment A wide spectrum vaccination programme against respiratory disease may reduce the horse's need to respond with this hyperplasia. Where pus is seen dripping from the swollen areas, treatment with antibiotics may be justified.

Prognosis Good. The condition usually disappears with time, and does not recur.

Pleurisy

Symptoms Breathing is rapid but shallow, and clearly painful. The horse has a fever.

Cause Pleurisy is due to an infection between the outer surface of the lungs and the inner chest wall. It is usually associated with a bacterial pneumonia and abscesses.

Treatment Any pus present in the chest cavity needs to be withdrawn. Intensive antibiotic therapy follows.

Prognosis Guarded to poor.

Rhinopneumonitis

Symptoms Rhinopneumonitis causes coughing, usually a more moist cough than with equine influenza. Perhaps because of the success of influenza vaccines, rhinopneumonitis is probably the commonest infectious cause of coughing in horses. Horses also develop a rather clear nasal discharge and possibly swollen lymph glands. In severe cases, affected mares may abort, often without showing marked respiratory symptoms *(Fig. 55)*.

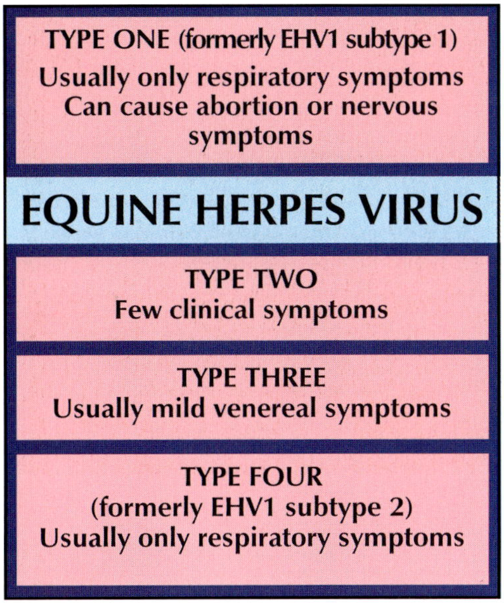

Fig. 55 The members of the Herpes family of viruses in the horse.

Cause Equine herpes viruses; both EHV1 and EHV4 viruses can cause respiratory symptoms, although EHV1 virus more commonly causes abortion and neurological symptoms.

Treatment There is no treatment to kill the virus. Bronchodilators, such as clenbuterol, and mucolytics will help to limit the effects on the lungs, and so decrease the chances of exercise-induced pulmonary haemorrhage in later years. There are now conventional vaccines available to control both respiratory and abortion symptoms, although so far there is not a single vaccine which has been proved to control both aspects of EHV. Experimentally, ISCOM (Immune Stimulating Complex) vaccines have also shown an ability to give some protection against the respiratory form of the disease.

Prognosis A very infectious disease which usually only causes mild symptoms. EIPH may recur in later years after an infection.

Sinusitis

Symptoms The primary symptom is a purulent nasal discharge which is usually only discharging from one nostril. Tapping the skull over the fluid-filled sinus gives a different sound from that over a normal, air-filled sinus. X-rays will show which sinus is affected.

Cause Usually a problem with the root of one of the upper molar teeth, which extend into the sinuses.

Treatment First, the basic cause has to be removed, primarily by removing damaged teeth. The sinus is then washed out using water and/or antiseptics through a hole drilled through the skull into the sinus.

Prognosis If treatment is continued long enough, recovery is usually complete.

Soft palate displacement

Symptoms The horse suddenly starts to make loud gurgling noises during fast exercise and pulls itself up. The noises then decreases and the horse can continue as if nothing has happened. In fact the horse's larynx has been pulled backwards, allowing the soft palate to move over (rather than under) the epiglottis and block the horse's airway. The condition is sometimes therefore referred to as 'swallowing the tongue'.

Cause The movement is due to an abnormal pull in the muscles which attach the larynx to the lower neck. It may well be that this pull is the result of an increased need for air because of some underlying lung problem.

Treatment If an underlying cause can be found, which reduces overall respiratory efficiency and so stimulates more forceful inspiration, this obviously needs treatment. Tying the horse's tongue tightly to its lower jaw during a race may prevent the larynx being pulled back. More permanently a section of the neck muscles may be removed surgically, allowing them to heal with a scar which effectively lengthens them. This reduces the force with which they can pull on the larynx.

Prognosis Once affected, the horse tends to continue to 'swallow its tongue' when galloped flat out, e.g. at the climax of a race.

Strangles

Symptoms Affected horses go off their food and have a raised temperature of around 104°F (40°). They have a nasal discharge which soons becomes purulent *(Fig. 56)*. Although the high temperature may drop after a couple of days, it then goes up again as the lymph nodes around the jaw and throat become swollen *(Figs. 57 & 58)*. Abscesses in these glands may burst, discharging thick pus. Strangles is usually a disease of young horses, when they are mixed together. It can reach epidemic proportions.

Cause The bacterium *Streptococcus equi*.

Treatment Disagreement exists over when antibiotic treatment should be started, because of the suggestion that with antibiotic therapy abscesses are more likely to become walled off from surrounding tissues. Treatment may therefore be delayed until after any abscesses in the lymph nodes have burst. When antibiotics are employed, penicillin is the drug usually used. Anti-inflammatory drugs may help to prevent the swollen abscesses making breathing difficult. Large abscesses may need to be lanced. There are no vaccines available in the UK, and their use elsewhere is controversial but widespread.

Prognosis Sometimes abscesses form in internal lymph glands (so-called bastard strangles) and cause bouts of colic etc. Purpura haemorrhagica (see page 139) can follow infections of strangles.

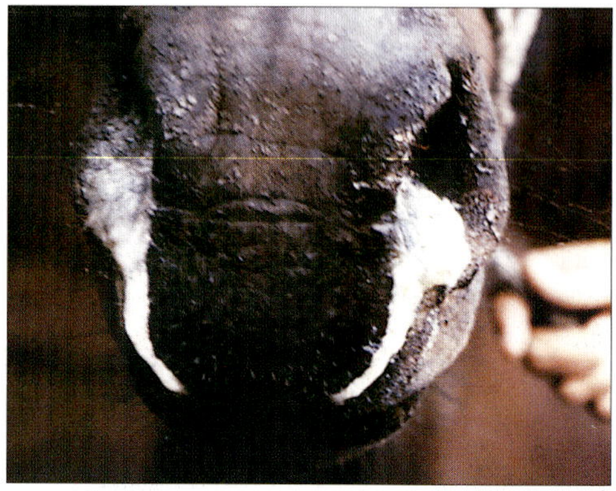

Fig. 56 *A horse with strangles*
The thick discharge from both nostrils comes from abscesses which have ruptured internally.

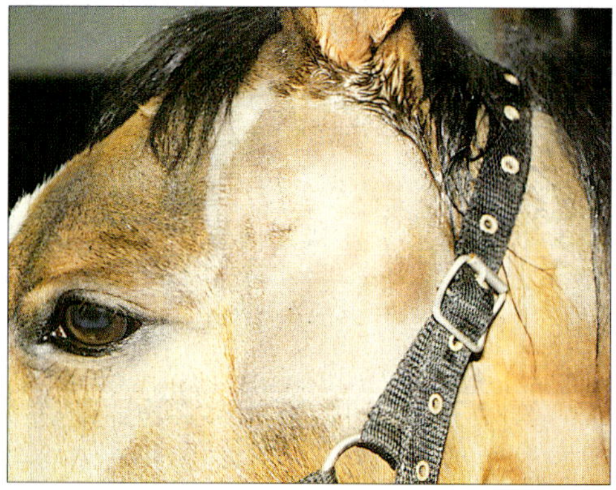

Fig. 57 A strangles abscess down the posterior border of the jaw.

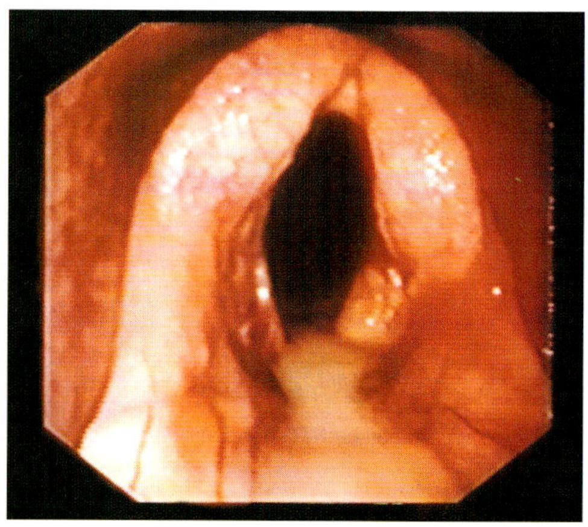

Fig. 58 Endoscopic view of a horse's larynx, showing pus as a result of strangles.

Tuberculosis

Symptoms Thankfully, tuberculosis is now exceedingly rare in horses in the developed world. Affected animals lose weight over a period. They may develop pneumonia, although the disease is usually centred in the intestine.

Cause The *Mycobacterium* family of bacteria, which affect both mammals and birds.

Treatment As a danger to human health, affected animals should be slaughtered.

Prognosis Untreated, this is a chronic, often fatal disease.

5: Diseases of the central nervous system and sensory organs

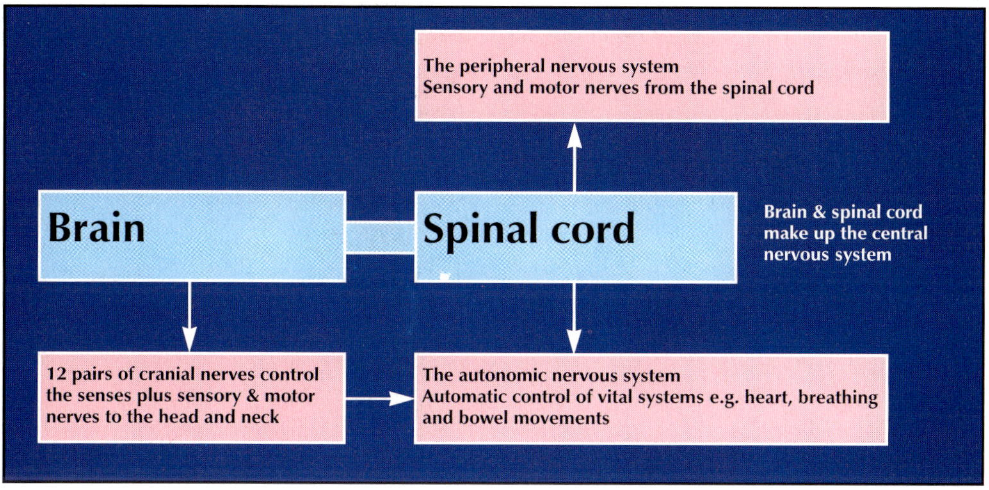

Fig. 59 *The organisation of the horse's nervous system*

There are marked similarities between the central nervous system and the cardiovascular system. In the latter, one system (the veins) returns blood to the heart and another (the arteries) channels the blood away from the heart; similarly, the central nervous system (CNS) has two distinct kinds of nerves connected to the brain, which occupies the central role in the nervous system in the same way that the heart does in the circulatory system *(Fig. 59)*. Nerve fibres are either sensory, transmitting information to the brain, or motor, transmitting messages from the brain to the muscles in order to carry out the brain's wishes.

The brain has three sections, carrying out different functions. The forebrain controls hormonal secretion within the body, mainly via the pituitary gland which lies just underneath it. The midbrain is concerned with sight and smell and the conscious voluntary control of movement, breathing and behaviour. The hindbrain is concerned with the automatic involuntary control of movement, breathing and behaviour.

There are twelve pairs of cranial nerves, which control the head, and deal with such vital functions as sight and hearing, as well as swallowing and aspects of breathing. The tenth cranial nerve, the vagus, has a very widespread role because it is involved with the autonomic nervous system, which comprises the para-sympathetic and sympathetic nervous systems. These are the systems which automatically control the bodily functions essential for life, such as heart rate, bowel movement and glandular secretions. Unlike the sensory and motor functions, these are not under conscious control.

Extending down from the brain is the spinal cord, which is protected by a bony

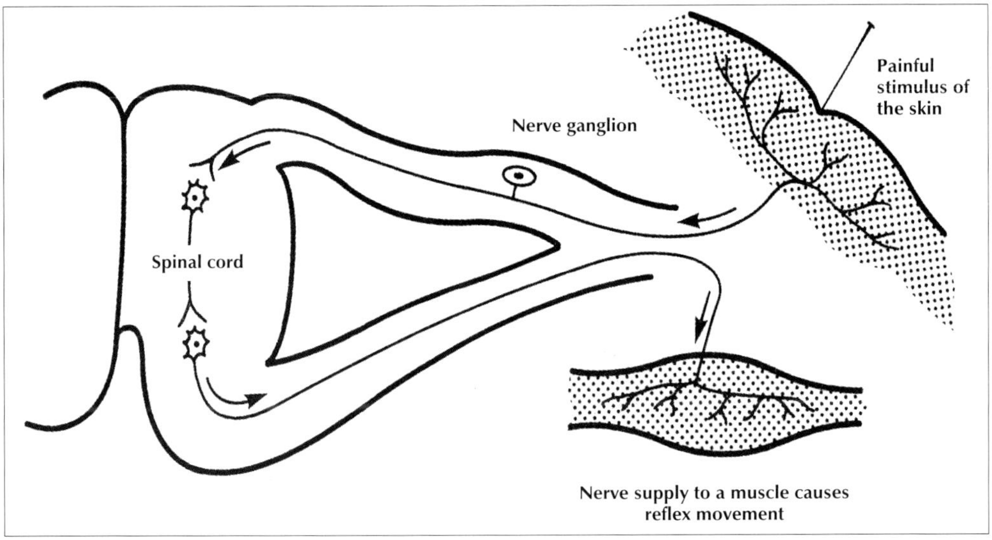

Fig. 60 *The spinal reflex arc*

structure, the vertebral column. Whereas the skull protecting the brain is a single structure, the vertebral column is made up of many individual bones called vertebrae. A pair of spinal nerves leaves the spinal cord between each pair of adjacent vertebrae. These then branch to supply both sensory and motor nerves to a particular area of the body. In man the spinal cord is often damaged by pressure from the intervertebral discs. These discs act as cushions between vertebrae but can be pushed upwards against the spinal cord. This does not happen in the horse, where disc problems are almost unknown.

A nerve is made up of many individual nerve cells or fibres. Each nerve cell has either a sensory role—passing messages to the brain and spinal cord (often called the central nervous system)—or a motor role—transmitting impulses to muscle cells. Cells never serve both functions. A nerve fibre may be several metres long, with a single nucleus surrounded by the cell body. Collections of nerve cell bodies form swellings along the nerve, called ganglia. These function as relays. When a nerve passes on its impulses to the next nerve in the chain, the fibre splits into many fine strands, called dendrites. These link with those of the adjoining fibre, but the message is actually carried across the gap, or synapse, between the dendrites by chemical transmitters.

Not all nerve impulses pass up the spinal cord to the brain. There are certain automatic reflex arcs built into the system. When a specific stimulus such as pain stimulates one end of a particular nerve fibre the message at the spinal cord 'short circuits' and sends out a pre-programmed message without waiting to hear what the brain has to say *(Fig. 60)*. If you prick a horse's leg with a needle, the horse will immediately pull its leg away. The speed of this reflex action is due to the fact that it is not necessary to wait until the message has travelled up to the horse's brain and back before a response is seen. A message goes to the brain, though, and the brain can, if it wants to, override the reflex action.

As the spinal cord approaches the brain, there are more nerve fibres because more nerves are joining the cable. So, damage to the spinal cord in one area can have a drastic effect on a part of the body which is anatomically a distance away but whose nerve fibres pass through the damaged area. Nerves are very sensitive cells. They operate by transmitting an electrical impulse along their long thin body.

Almost any damage to an individual cell prevents it from transmitting impulses. The nearer to the brain or spinal cord the damage occurs, the wider the area which is affected. If a horse breaks its neck it will almost certainly be paralysed from the neck downwards. Remember, however, that it might still be alive because breathing and circulation control is carried out via the vagus nerve which does not run down the vertebral column.

The nerve fibres need to be surrounded by an insulating layer which performs the same function as the plastic covering on an electrical wire. Minute electrical impulses pass along nerve fibres and these must not be allowed to trigger every muscle along their path. So the peripheral nerves have a sheath of a fat-like substance called myelin. Any injury or chemical substance which damages that myelin sheath interferes with the efficiency of the nerve function. The central nervous system, the brain and spinal cord, has a slightly different system. The nervous tissue of the brain is completely surrounded by fluid, and this fluid is contained by membranes called the meninges. This system protects the nervous tissue from trauma of various kinds.

Damage to the nervous system shows itself in two ways. Paralysis is a complete relaxation of all the muscles supplied by a particular motor nerve, caused by damage that prevents any impulses passing along that nerve. So a paralysed leg, for example, hangs down limply and cannot be moved. Similar damage to a sensory nerve causes a complete loss of sensation over the area supplied by the nerve. We make use of this when carrying out nerve blocks. Injecting a small volume of local anaesthetic around a nerve prevents impulses passing, and so prevents the horse feeling any sensation in the area supplied. The other response of the nervous system to injury is to send a continuous impulse down a motor nerve. As a result the muscle supplied contracts and stays contracted. This is the situation that occurs, for example, in tetanus with the well-known result that the jaws can be locked shut.

The eye

The horse's eye has the same anatomical structure as the human eye *(Fig. 61)*. The eyeball itself is almost spherical (it bulges slightly at the front) and is very tough. The disc at the front, where the eyeball is transparent, is called the cornea. Light passes through the cornea to the lens and then to the inside surface of the eye, which is largely covered with a layer of light-sensitive cells, called the retina.

There are two control mechanisms in the eye. The iris is the coloured part which we see when we look at an eye. It contains muscles which can enlarge or decrease the size of the hole (pupil) through which light passes into the eye. It does so in response to varying degreees of brightness. In the dark the pupil opens

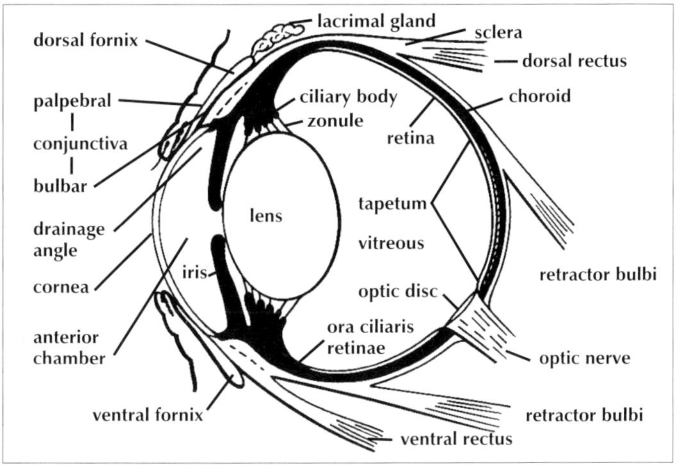

Fig. 61 *The structure of the horse's eye*

very wide and in bright sunlight it closes up, or constricts. Hanging from the iris are often seen small black bodies called corpora nigra. Their function is unknown. The lens is immediately behind the pupil and is suspended by muscles which provide the second form of control. When these muscles contract or relax, the lens becomes thicker or thinner. In this way the eye can focus light from varying distances on to the retina.

The sensitive retina contains two distinct types of nerve cells, rods and cones. However we know little, if anything, about what the horse can or cannot see. Fibres from the retina meet at the so-called optic disc, where the optic nerve emerges from the back of the eye.

The eye has a number of muscles attached to the outside of the sclera, the tough white layer of the eyeball, and these control the movement of the eye. It is important to realise that the horse's eyes are in a fundamentally different position from our own. Our eyes are on the front of our head and are directed frontwards. Their fields of vision overlap to a large extent, providing the 3-D vision which enables us, for instance, to appreciate fine detail on objects. The horse's eyes, on the other hand are set high up on the side of its head. The horse therefore looks forward out of the corner of its eye, and there is very little overlap between the two fields of view to provide binocular vision. Vision to the side and rear is, however, much better than in man. When the horse evolved on the plains, it was obviously an advantage for it to be able to see through almost 360° without moving its head, as this meant that predators could not creep up in a blind spot. The relative unimportance of binocular vision to the horse explains why horses that have lost the use of one eye are often still able to judge distances and jump, even at speed.

The horse's eye is protected by eyelids, the muscles of which are incredibly strong. Anyone who has tried to forcibly prise them open will know how strong the eyelid muscles are, and how quickly they can react and close the eye.

Other senses

The nerve endings which are responsible for the sense of smell are scattered over the membrane which lines the nasal passages. Horses have a good sense of smell, which can detect sex hormones in urine passed by other horses. Horses also have a good sense of hearing. Their ear has a similar structure to ours. The inner ear consists of a series of fluid-filled tubes that are responsible for balance. The middle ear is actually responsible for hearing. It is separated from the external ear by the eardrum, but it has an opening to the pharynx at the back of the mouth via a tube called the eustachian tube (see page 39). A special feature in the horse is the fact that each eustachian tube widens into a large membranous sac called the guttural pouch (see page 39). This is situated just under the skin below the ear. The external ear canal ends at the pinna, the large sound funnel which forms the external ear. The pinna can be moved around in order to judge the direction from which a sound has come.

Botulism

Symptoms The first sign is usually paralysis of the muscles involved in chewing and swallowing. The horse stands over its food and water, but they just drop out of its mouth. As more nerves become involved, the legs weaken and eventually the horse cannot stand. Death is due to paralysis of the muscles involved in breathing.

Cause The disease is often the result of the horse eating food contaminated with toxin from the *Clostridium botulinum* bacteria, rather than the bacterium itself. 'Big Bale Silage' has proved particularly dangerous because if incorrectly stored or handled it can provide ideal conditions for the growth of the bacteria in dead rodents, and so on, inside the bale.

Treatment Antitoxin can be used to counteract the toxin. Large doses of penicillin will kill any bacteria present.

Prognosis The quicker the onset of the symptoms, the more likely the horse is to die. If it becomes unable to stand, complications such as pneumonia may set in and cause death.

Cataracts

Symptoms There are usually no symptoms visible to the naked eye. With the aid of an ophthalmoscope, areas of opacity can be seen in the lens of the eye. These vary in position and size. Only if they involve almost the whole of the lens is the horse likely to be obviously blind. It must be appreciated, however, that relatively small cataracts in the centre of the lens may cause problems when bright light makes the horse close its pupil.

Cause Cataracts can be present in foals from birth *(Fig. 62)*. Periodic ophthalmia (see page 61), may result in cataract formation, and they can also develop after eye injuries. Cataracts do not usually develop as a result of old age in the horse.

Treatment By and large, no treatment is given. Surgical removal of cataracts is possible in the horse, but is usually only contemplated when the cataracts are obviously interfering with vision and when there is no evidence of any other eye problem.

Prognosis Cataracts do not usually go away. They may well, on the other hand, progress and involve even more of the lens. It is not considered a good practice to breed from a horse which had congenital cataracts at birth, although it is safe to do so from a horse which developed a cataract later in life.

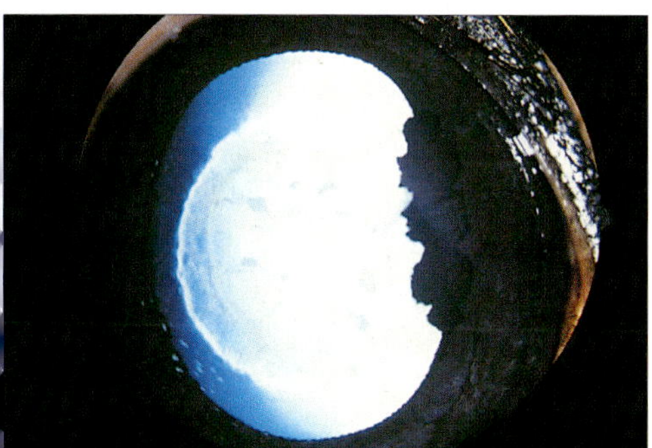

Fig. 62 A cataract in a foal's eye.

Conjunctivitis

Symptoms The skin around the affected eye is puffed out as a result of the swelling of the conjunctiva, or sensitive membranes around the eye *(Fig. 63)*. The eyelids may be partly or completely closed. There is usually a discharge from the eye. At first this will be clear, but within a day or two it will become opaque and pussy as bacterial infection becomes established.

Cause Some sort of trauma is necessary to cause the initial inflammation, which subsequently becomes secondarily infected. Squamous cell carcinomas may affect the conjunctiva *(Fig. 64)*.

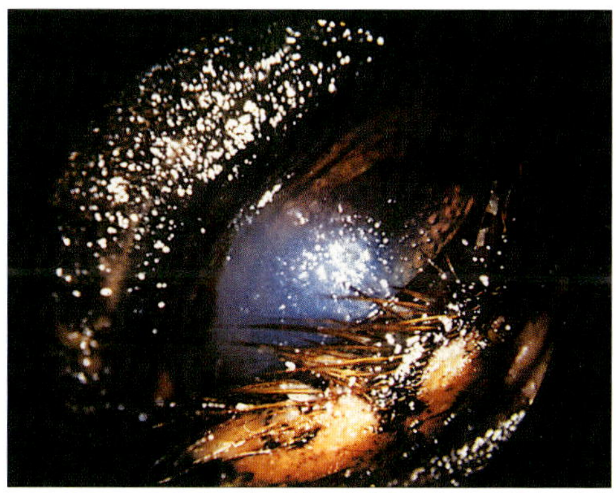

Fig. 63 *Conjuctivitis*
The sensitive pink membranes around the eye are swollen and inflamed.

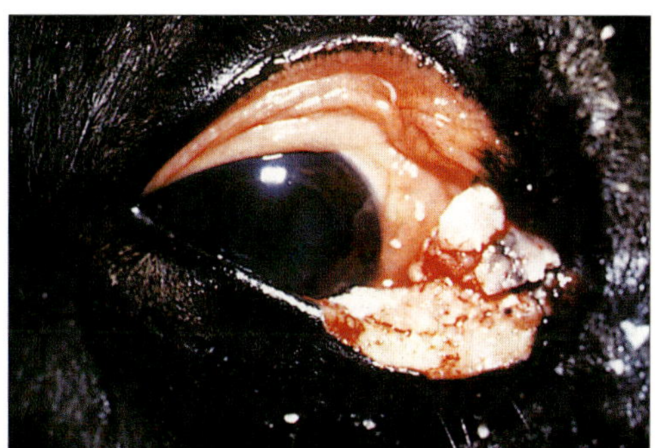

Fig. 64 Squamous cell carcinoma.

Treatment The drugs used will depend on what damage, if any, has been caused to the actual eyeball. Cortisone will reduce the swelling and inflammation quite quickly. It is usually combined with an antibiotic to kill the infection.

Prognosis Good.

Corneal wounds

Symptoms Part or all of the front (usually transparent) surface of the eye becomes opaque and bluish-white. The eye may be obviously painful, causing the horse to repeatedly rub its head. The pink membranes lining the eyelids, the conjunctiva, may be swollen and inflamed. With time bright red blood vessels may be seen in the cornea, moving from the outside towards the seat of the injury. If the surface of the cornea is broken, it will attract the dye, fluorescein, which is put into the eye in order to detect such wounds and show their extent.

Cause There are three main causes of corneal injury. Damage by a blunt object may merely cause general bruising. Damage by a sharp object may actually penetrate the surface of the cornea, possibly causing an ulcer. Damage by a foreign body may be a continuous process because small foreign bodies, such as the husks of grass and cereal seeds, become fixed to the surface of the cornea. When this happens they may be almost invisible.

Treatment A distinction has to be made as to whether the surface of the cornea has been destroyed or not. If it hasn't, then corticosteroids can be used to reduce the inflammation. They are always combined with an antibiotic to fight any infection present. If the corneal surface has been partially removed, then corticosteroids cannot be used because they delay the healing of such ulcerated areas.

Antibiotics alone may then be used. Atropine may help to ensure that deeper parts of the eye do not develop adhesions by dilating the pupil. Whenever using ointments or drops in the eye treatment must be repeated four to six times a day because they are washed away by tears.

Prognosis Good, although chronic ulcers may require cautery.

Crib biting

Symptoms The horse bites at fixed objects such as the edge of the stable door or grasps an object in its teeth for hours a day, often causing great damage to its surroundings in the process. The front edges of both upper and lower incisor teeth become worn away *(Fig. 65)*. As a result, cursory inspection of the horse's teeth may indicate that the individual is older than it really is.

Cause Probably boredom. The horse appears to obtain pleasure from the act, and it may be that it causes the release of endorphins (natural morphine-like substances) into its bloodstream.

Treatment Smearing noxious substances on likely objects may reduce crib biting.

Prognosis Once the vice is established, it is extremely difficult to break. Affected horses may progress to wind suck.

Eastern equine encephalitis

Symptoms The principal symptoms are fever and brain damage. The horse may grind its teeth or press its head against the wall. It may go around in circles or become blind. Eventually paralysis sets in, and the horse becomes unable to stand.

Cause A virus that is transmitted by mosquitoes. It is commonest down the eastern seaboard of North and South America.

Treatment There is no specific medication. Vaccines are available.

Prognosis The disease is often fatal. Recovered horses may have some brain damage, and are often called 'dummies'.

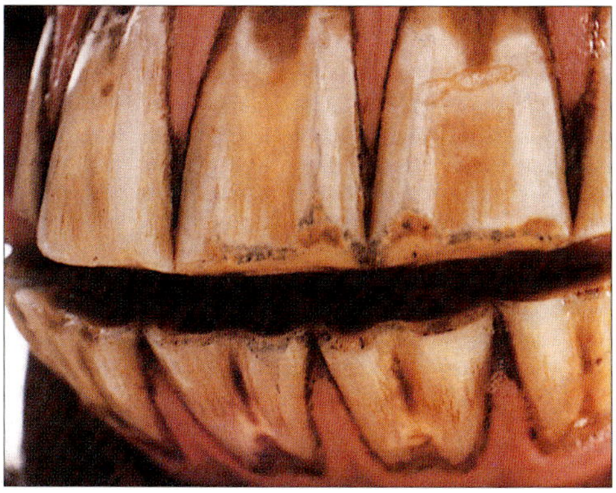

Fig. 65 *A front view of a crib biter's incisor teeth* Note how the front edges are worn away.

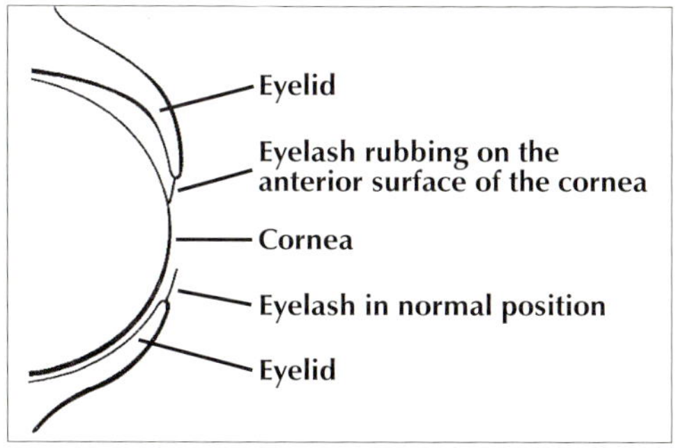

Fig. 66 *Entropion*

Entropion

Symptoms Inflammation of one or both eyes, with increased production of tears. The edge of the eyelid is turned inwards, so that the eyelashes rub on the eyeball.

Cause This may be a congenital condition in foals. In older horses it can be a temporary problem resulting from swelling of the eyelid *(Fig. 66)*.

Treatment The eyelid must be prevented from turning inwards. Temporary stitches may hold it away from the eyeball. A more permanent cure requires the removal of a small fold of skin from the affected eyelid.

Prognosis Recurrence is unlikely after surgery.

Equine degenerative myeloencephalopathy

Symptoms Hind leg weakness or ataxia in horses less than 3 years old.

Cause Many cases are associated with vitamin E deficiency.

Treatment Increased vitamin E levels in diet reduces the incidence.

Prognosis Poor.

Equine protozoal myeloencephalitis

Symptoms A variety of nervous symptoms can occur although lameness is often the first indication. Commonest during warm weather.

Cause A coccidian parasite, *Sarcocystis,* invades the central nervous system.

Treatment Pyrimethamine and trimethoprim sulphadiazine are given in combination.

Prognosis Poor. Relapses are common even if the horse improves with treatment.

Facial paralysis

Symptoms Paralysis of the muscles of the lips results in one or both of the lips on the affected side hanging loosely. This may affect the horse's ability to eat. The horse may make an abnormal noise at exercise due to an effect on the false nostril (a fold of skin just inside the nostril).

Cause The condition is usually due to a blow on the face. It can occur as a result of pressure on a nerve while a horse is recumbent, e.g. under anaesthetic. It can also appear with no known cause.

Treatment Time is usually the only treatment. The mouth should be checked for any food accumulations. Steroids may help reduce inflammation after a blow.

Prognosis Guarded. Recovery may take months rather than days.

Head shaking

Symptoms The horse shakes its head violently when ridden, usually in a vertical direction. As a result it may become unrideable. The head shaking is usually only present during summer, ceasing once the frosty weather starts. It is often worse in conditions when the air is still and humid. Similarly the horse may shake its head more when ridden close to a hedgerow than when out in the middle of a large field.

Cause Many individual causes have been diagnosed, but usually no cause is found. Although the symptoms worsen in conditions which encourage flies and midges, all efforts to prove a link have been unsuccessful. There is now evidence that the problem is often an allergic rhinitis (inflammation of the lining of the nasal passages).

Treatment A specific cause diagnosed during a thorough examination must be treated. Where the cause is undiagnosed, wearing a fly fringe over the eyes or nose may reduce the amount of head shaking. Surgical cutting of the infraorbital nerve may relieve the symptoms.

Prognosis The affected horse will always be so, at least during summer. The head shaking may become more pronounced in time.

Hepatic encephalopathy

Symptoms Sleepiness and lethargy. The horse may become blind and stand pressing its head against a wall *(Fig. 67)* or stagger around unaware of its surroundings. Liver enzymes in the blood may be raised. It may be jaundiced.

Cause The condition can be the result of any severe liver disease (see page 73).

Treatment If possible, have the initial cause of liver damage treated. Vitamin B injections combined with a high carbohydrate/low protein diet may help.

Prognosis Poor.

Herpes myeloencephalitis

Symptoms A lack of coordination (notably of the hind legs) shortly after exposure to equine herpes type 1 virus. Paralysis may set in.

Cause A particularly virulent strain of the equine herpes type 1 virus attacks the nerves as well as, or instead of, the respiratory system with which the virus is so commonly linked (see page 51).

Treatment There is no treatment to kill the virus. Nursing care is vital to prevent the horse from injuring itself while staggering, and to prevent pressure sores if the horse is recumbent. A vaccine against EHV1 is now available.

Prognosis Many horses recover completely. If they become recumbent, however, and unable to stand up, they may die from complications such as pneumonia.

Microphthalmia

Symptoms The foal is born with one eye very much reduced in size, usually about the size of a pea *(Fig. 68)*. The small eyeball does not function. The eye socket may not be correspondingly reduced in size, and so relatively large amounts of the conjunctiva are visible around the eye, especially the third eyelid.

Cause The condition is congenital.

Treatment None possible or necessary.

Prognosis It is probably not advisable to breed from affected animals.

Neuritis of the cauda equina

Symptoms Progressive paralysis of the tail and the sphincter muscles controlling the rectum and the urethra. As a result the horse may show colic because of a failure to pass faeces, and the skin of the hind legs becomes scalded by urine dribbling out of the vagina or the prepuce. In time the hind leg muscles become affected as the weakness spreads. Sometimes the facial nerves may also be involved. It is not known why the nerves supplying the tail and rectum degenerate first.

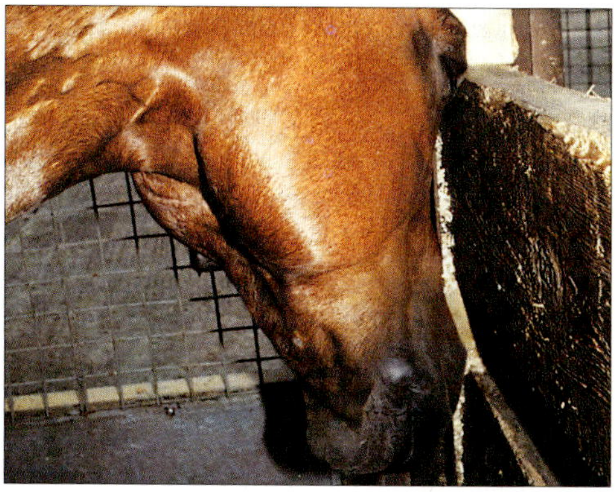

Fig. 67 Head pressing as a result of hepatic encephalopathy.

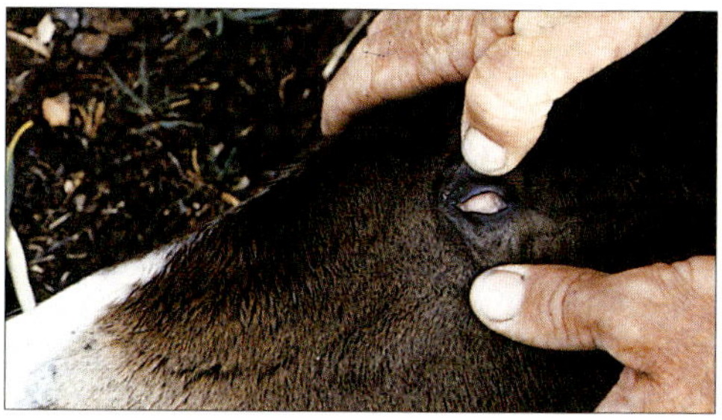

Fig. 68 Microphthalmia in a newborn foal.

Causes The condition is thought to be due to the horse becoming immune to its own tissues, in particular the nerve cells.

Treatment There is no treatment.

Prognosis Poor. Death is usually the result of prolonged recumbency, cystitis or colic.

Periodic ophthalmia

Symptoms This condition gets its name from the fact that the symptoms, inflammatory changes in the eye, flare up and then disappear only to reappear at a later date. During the periods of remission the eyes may appear completely normal. When the disease is active, one or both eyes are very inflamed and painful. The membranes around the eye may be swollen, and the eye may appear milky white (hence the name 'moon blindness') due to inflammation of the cornea. The pupil is usually constricted. With successive attacks, the horse often becomes completely blind as the internal structures of the eye become permanently damaged.

Cause Periodic ophthalmia appears to be due to a localised allergic reaction. The bacteria Leptospira and the parasite Onchocerca are just two of the causes which have been implicated, but in many cases no cause has been pinpointed.

Treatment Ivermectin is given to eliminate any Onchocerca present. The allergic symptoms are relieved by steroid injections into the conjunctival membranes around the eye. Antibiotics treat any secondary bacterial infections, and Leptospira, if present. Atropine helps to keep the pupil dilated. Because affected horses are sensitive to light, they are best kept in a darkened loosebox.

Prognosis The disease is usually progressive, and even when caught in the early stages may result in blindness.

Rabies

Symptoms The initial symptoms are very variable, but after a period when it is hyper-excitable, the horse becomes dull. As its vocal cords become paralysed the horse may have a very changed whinny. It will not drink. Eventually, paralysis of the hindquarters leads to collapse and death.

Cause The rabies virus can affect all mammals. The horse becomes infected from saliva when bitten by a rabid animal or bat. Horses rarely pass the virus on to other horses or animals.

Treatment There is no treatment. Prevention is possible via annual vaccination, although this is not permitted in the UK, where rabies does not occur.

Prognosis Affected horses will die.

Radial paralysis

Symptoms One of the forelegs hangs limply down from the body. It feels no sensation, and the horse is unable to control its movement, especially forward.

Cause Pressure during recumbency for

surgery or a blow to the front of the shoulder, where the radial nerve is relatively exposed.

Treatment There is no treatment.

Prognosis With sufficient time the nerves often recover.

Stringhalt
Symptoms The horse picks up one or both of its hind legs in a very exaggerated way when it walks or goes backwards.

Cause Unknown, although in Australia it is often associated with plant toxins.

Treatment Cutting the lateral digital extensor tendon may cure the condition.

Prognosis Guarded.

Sweeny (suprascapular paralysis)
Symptoms The muscles of the shoulder atrophy. The horse has an abnormal gait, 'shoulder slip', as the shoulder is moved.

Cause A blow to the shoulder can cause the damage. In draught horses it can be due to pressure from an ill-fitting collar.

Treatment Rest prevents further stretching of the nerve by abnormal gait. Initially, steroids may reduce inflammation around the nerve. Surgery to free scar tissue around the nerve can be performed three weeks after the injury.

Prognosis Guarded.

Tetanus
Symptoms The main symptom is a muscular spasm. When this affects the muscles of the jaw, it produces lockjaw. Spasm of the leg muscles make walking difficult, or even impossible. The spasms may visibly worsen as a result of sudden sounds or movements. Raising the horse's head often causes its third eyelid to be pulled across from the inner corner of its eye.

Cause Spores of the bacterium *Clostridium tetani* can only become active in dying tissue which is not exposed to any oxygen, such as a deep, penetrating wound. Because the organism is common in soil, any wound may allow the spores to enter the horse's body. The bacteria produce a toxin which affects the nerves.

Treatment An antitoxin can counteract some of the effect of the toxin. Meanwhile penicillin and cleaning of any visible wounds may kill the bacterium itself. Often it is a question of keeping the horse alive by intensive nursing long enough for it to recover. A toxoid vaccine (a vaccine against the toxin) is available.

Prognosis Recovery to complete normality may take weeks or months.

Transit tetany
Symptoms Horses sweat and develop muscle twitches. Later they become unsteady and uncoordinated. They collapse and eventually die in convulsions.

Cause Stress, often associated with transit or endurance rides, combined with low levels of blood magnesium and calcium. Mares suckling foals are susceptible as they are losing calcium in the milk. The condition is then called lactation tetany.

Treatment Intravenous infusions of magnesium and calcium can reverse the condition, especially in the early stages.

Prognosis Good with treatment as long as the stress is removed.

Venezuelan equine encephalitis
Symptoms, Cause, Treatment and Prognosis: Similar to those of eastern equine encephalitis (page 58).

Western equine encephalitis
Symptoms Similar to those of eastern equine encephalitis (page 58).

Cause The causative virus lives in wild birds in western North America. It is spread to horses by mosquitoes, which can also spread the disease to humans.

Treatment Vaccines are available.

Prognosis Unless paralysis sets in, good for recovery.

Wind sucking

Symptoms The horse arches its neck and pulls its larynx out of the normal position for breathing so that it protrudes through the soft palate (often by grasping a fixed object with its teeth; see crib biting page 58). It then swallows air into its stomach. There is no scientific evidence that this causes digestive problems. It does, however, cause considerable noise, especially around feeding time when the vice tends to be more frequent. Affected horses may cause considerable damage to fencing etc.

Cause Possibly boredom. The horse appears to obtain pleasure from the act of swallowing air, and horses often develop the vice after watching affected horses wind sucking.

Treatment The vice may be prevented, especially in the early stages, by fixing a specially shaped 'yoke' behind the larynx so that the horse can breathe but not swallow *(Fig. 69)*. In extreme cases surgery to cut the nerves and muscles which enable the horse to retract its larynx may work.

Prognosis Once this vice is established, it is extremely difficult to break. After surgery horses may continue to crib bite.

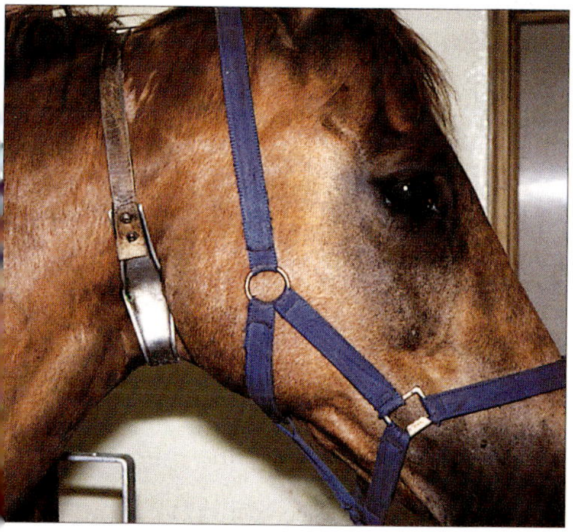

Fig. 69 *The use of a wind sucking strap*

Wobbler syndrome

Symptoms Affected horses appear unsteady on their legs, notably the hind legs. These may appear stiff, not bending as much as normal. The basic problem is that the horse is not fully aware of the exact positioning of its hind legs. Walking the horse backwards or in circles may exaggerate its unsteadiness, as may walking it downhill or with its head raised. It is often far easier than normal to push the horse's hindquarters down, or to make the horse sway as it walks by pulling sideways on its tail. The symptoms appear in yearlings and two year olds. They may occur suddenly or there may be a gradual deterioration.

Cause Pressure on the spinal cord due to an injury, or abnormal growth and shaping of the individual vertebrae on the neck of the growing horse. The first five or six neck vertebrae are usually afflicted. Symptoms may affect anywhere behind this because any of the messages to and from the brain may be affected.

Treatment Radical surgery has been attempted in the USA, where the spinal cord changes appear usually to involve different vertebrae from those involved in the UK. The success rate in terms of producing a horse capable of work is not good. Corticosteroids may give some improvement as they reduce the inflammation caused in the membranes around the spinal cord. Affected foals may recover with restricted diet and exercise, allowing the growing vertebrae to correct the problem.

Prognosis There is so little chance of the horse being able to undertake exercise that euthanasia is often the only course.

6:The digestive system

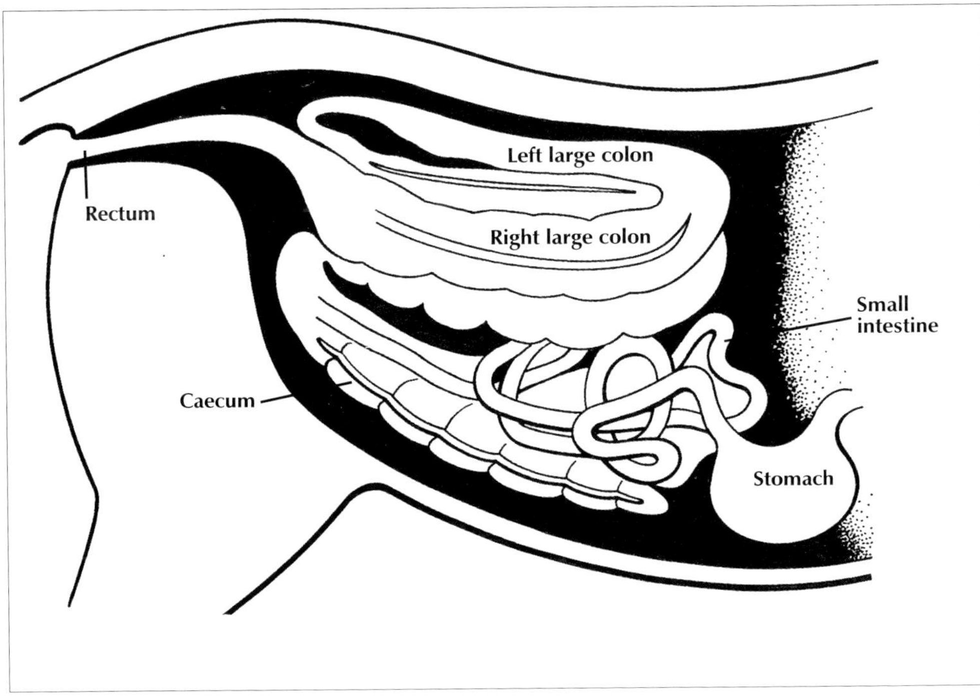

Fig. 70 *The horse's digestive system*

The alimentary tract is a tube which stretches from the horse's mouth to its rectum. Along the length of that tube are regions of specialisation which enable the horse to take in raw food (in the wild, grass and roughage, often supplemented by man with so-called short food such as oats) and to digest it to release the vital nutrients which the horse needs *(Fig. 70)*. The waste products are then passed out as faeces from the rectum. The horse's digestive system is a hybrid. It is a cross between a simple system such as is found in man, and the complicated four-stomach system found in other grass-eating animals such as cattle and sheep *(Fig. 71)*.

The first stage of digestion is to prepare the food. This involves chewing long fibres such as straw into smaller lengths and grinding grains such as oats into fragments. The chewed food is then mixed with saliva from the salivary glands. The horse only produces saliva when it is chewing. Saliva contains simple digestive enzymes which mark the start of the digestive process. As I mentioned earlier the horse naturally eats grass, which it cuts off in short lengths with its front incisor teeth. It is the development of these teeth, and their subsequent wear which we use to age a horse *(Fig 72)*. The horse does not use its canine teeth to tear flesh apart as a carnivore does. The small canine tooth in male horses is called … tush. The cheek teeth, or molars, are the chewing and grinding teeth, whilst the tongue acts as a large mixing rod which moves the food around and helps to mix …

	Stomach type	Ability to digest plant cellulose	Site of major bacterial digestion	Size of caecum
Man	Relatively large stomach	—	—	Small
Cow	Rumen, reticulum, omasum & abomasum	+	Rumen	—
Horse	Relatively small stomach	+	Large colon	Large

Fig. 71 *A comparison between the digestive systems of different animals*

well with the saliva.

From the mouth the food passes through a chamber called the pharynx, where the horse has to be careful that no food particles get through the larynx and into the respiratory system (see Chapter 4, page 39). Instead, the food is swallowed into the oesophagus, or gullet. This is a muscular tube which pushes the food down through the chest cavity to the stomach *(Fig. 73)*. Once the food enters the oesophagus the horse no longer has any control over its movement. The rest of the alimentary tract uses moving waves of alternate contraction and relaxation, called peristalsis, to move the contents along.

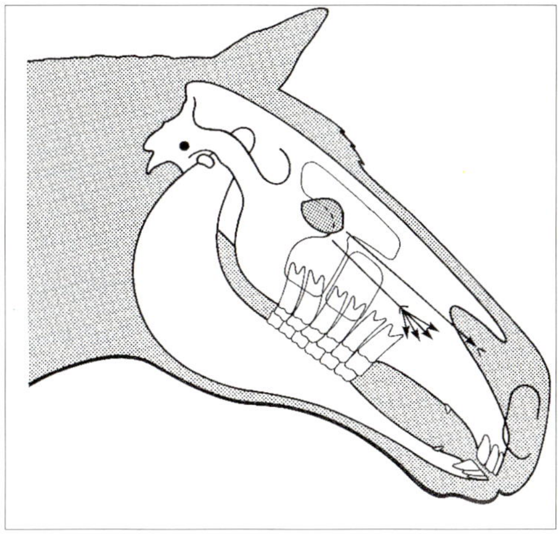

Fig. 72 *Diagram of the horse's skull and lower jaw,* showing incisor and molar teeth.

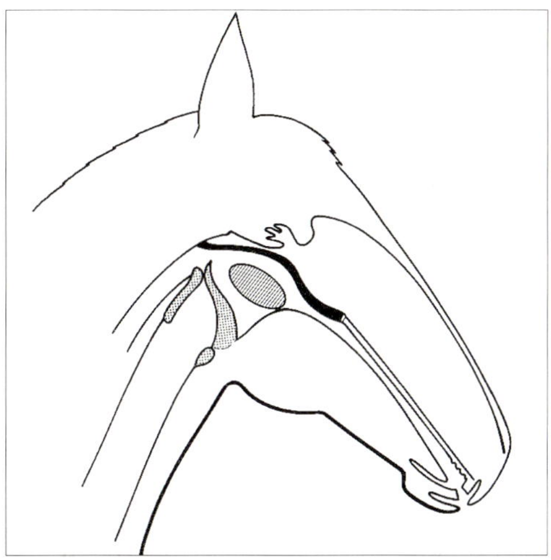

Fig. 73 *Diagram of a horse swallowing a bolus of food*
The epiglottis has blocked off the entrance to the trachea so no food goes down into the lungs. The food is just about to enter the oesophagus.

The horse's stomach is relatively small compared to that of other grass-eating animals. There is only a narrow entrance where the oesophagus joins the stomach, and this means that the horse cannot vomit up stomach contents except in extremis. Digestive enzymes are released by the stomach wall, breaking down the food material into simple nutrients which are absorbed by the small intestine.

The stomach contents are markedly acidic, which is helpful in the fight against infection. Many pathogenic bacteria cannot survive in this acidic environment, and so are killed off before they reach the intestines. It is during the food's passage along the approximately 22 metres (70 feet) of small intestine that the soluble carbohydrates (or starches) and most of the proteins are digested. The small intestine forms a series of U-shaped loops with a sheet of membrane, or mesentery, crossing the loops and attaching the intestine to the dorsal body wall. The blood supply to each loop of small intestine starts at the open end of the U, and radiates out like the spokes of a wheel to the intestine.

Grass and other plant material contains a substance called cellulose which mammalian digestive enzymes, including those of humans, cannot digest. Horses do so by utilising the digestive abilities of millions of bacteria and protozoa which live in the next section of the digestive tract, the large colon. The horse's large colon therefore fulfils a function rather like the rumen of the cow. The bacteria and protozoa which live there are completely independent of the horse but obtain their food source from the horse. In return they release simple carbohydrates and proteins which can be absorbed by the wall of the large colon.

The large colon has a relatively large diameter. It has an unusual shape because it is just like two U-shaped loops lying one on top of each and joined at one end. So there is a point where the large colon bends back on itself through 180° in order to start the second loop. This point is called the pelvic flexure. At the same spot the diameter drastically reduces in size. This is a common site of impaction for fibrous material. The walls of the large colon absorb water. Not just the water which the horse took in as food and drink, but also the water which was part of the saliva and digestive juices. The digested material therefore becomes much drier as it passes along the large colon, until eventually it is passed out of the rectum in the familiar form.

There is one other major part of the alimentary tract. This is the caecum. In human beings the caecum is a small insignificant structure, the appendix. In the horse it has a volume about twice that of the stomach. The caecum is a blind-ending sack which opens off the main alimentary tract at the junction between the small intestine and the large colon. It acts rather like a reservoir of intestinal contents for regulating flow and water absorption.

Colic

The symptoms of many of the diseases affecting the alimentary tract are very similar, and are usually referred to as the symptoms of colic. Colic is therefore a name for the symptoms of abdominal pain rather then a specific entity in itself. Pain may be caused by the stretching of the peritoneal membranes that cover all the abdominal organs. It can also be caused by distension of the muscles of the intestinal wall.

A horse with acute abdominal pain may be restless and keep looking around at its abdomen. Such pain is severe but not continuous. It may try to kick at its abdomen, or paw the ground with its front feet. The horse may keep lying down and often will repeatedly roll over from side to side *(Fig. 74)*. Sometimes a horse is driven frantic by the pain and will throw itself around without regard to the injuries it might cause itself. With more chronic pain, on the contrary, the horse may just lie down and remain very still. Such pain is less severe, but may well be continuous.

A horse with colic will often sweat, either all over its body or in patches over the shoulders, neck or hind quarters. The heart rate may be markedly increased, both as a result of the pain and as a result of the changes in the balance of fluids and electrolytes in the blood during major abdominal disturbances. Diagnosis of individual diseases can be made through studying the symtoms of colic *(Fig. 75)*.

When assessing a horse with colic,

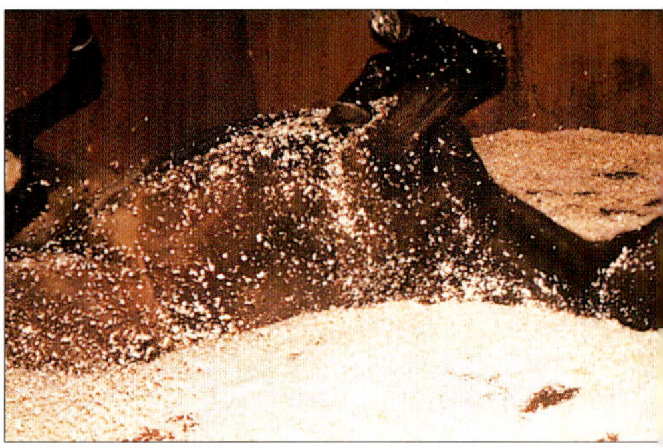

Fig. 74 A horse rolling with pain during colic.

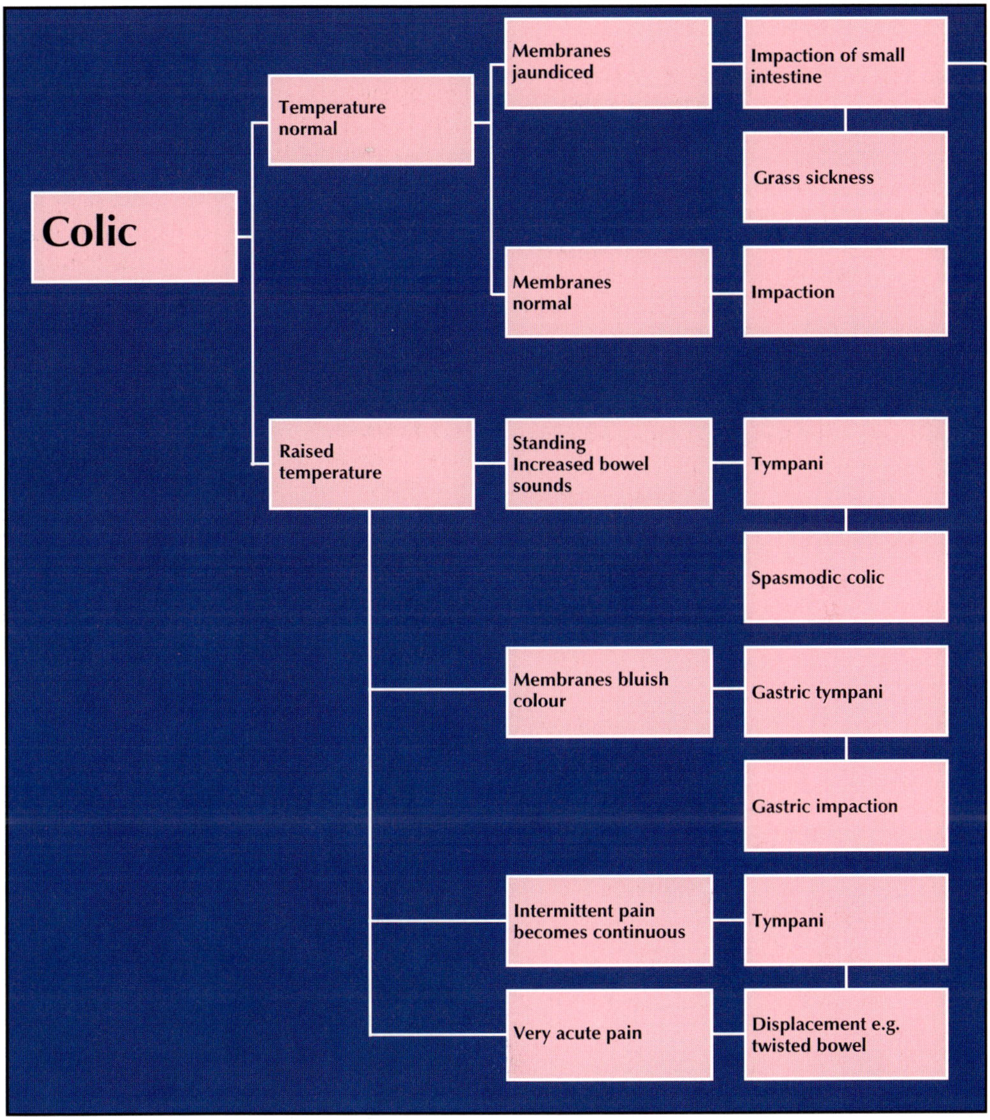

Fig. 75 *The different types of colic*

there are certain guidelines which have proved useful in indicating when the horse is seriously ill, and even possibly at risk of dying unless treatment is successful. A heart rate over 65 beats per minute is a warning sign. Even more serious is a capillary refill time of more than four seconds; this can be observed by pressing firmly on the mucous membrane of the horse's gums and then removing your finger. It is a serious sign if it takes more than four seconds for the capillaries to refill, and for the white mark you have made to return to its normal pink colour again. It is also a serious sign if the mucous membranes around the eyes become very congested and brick-red in colour.

With the disturbances in fluids and electrolytes during colic, the horse can become dehydrated. It may be possible to detect this by taking hold of a fold of skin over the neck and seeing whether the skin remains in a fold when you release it or whether it springs back flat almost immediately as it does in a healthy horse.

Veterinarians may assess this factor more accurately by taking a blood sample and measuring the horse's PCV (packed cell volume, see page 123). It is normally around 40%, but will be very much higher if the horse is dehydrated.

The liver

The liver is often dealt with as part of the digestive system although it is basically separate from the continuous tube of the alimentary tract. There is, however, a bile duct which leads from the liver to the intestines. Bile is produced in the liver and is a mixture of bile salts which help digestion (especially of fat) and bile pigments, the waste products of haemoglobin breakdown. The horse does not have a gall bladder to store bile because in nature the horse grazes continuously and needs a continuous flow of bile.

The liver consists of sheets of cells which are in contact with the blood circulation on one side and the bile ducts and channels on the other side. The liver cells convert sugars in the blood to a special starch called glycogen. Much of this glycogen is released back into the blood for transport to the muscles where it is stored as an energy source. The liver is therefore a vital organ without which the muscles cannot function. Thankfully the liver has very good powers of recuperation and so long term liver problems are rare in the horse. When they do arise it is often as a result of the liver's additional role in deactivating poisonous substances.

Jaundice—the development of a yellowish colour in the skin and the mucous membranes around the eyes and mouth—is due to some form of liver malfunction. The yellow colour is caused by the presence of bile pigment that has not been discharged down the bile duct into the intestines. This may be as a result of an obstruction of the bile ducts or it may be because more haemoglobin than the liver can deal with has been broken down. Both the fat of the horse and the mucous membranes of its mouth tend to be more yellow in colour than in other animals. As a result, jaundice is sometimes wrongly diagnosed in the horse unless proper blood samples are taken.

Feeding

The horse is a grazing animal. Even the largest hunter can obtain all its nutritional requirements from grass or from good quality hay as long as sufficient quantities are available. However, when a horse performs work, new nutritional requirements are stimulated. In all but the lightest work these requirements must be fuelled by concentrate feeding. As the horse is a grazing animal, its digestive tract is designed to cope with frequent small quantities of food rather than sudden large bucketsful.

Food is made up of carbohydrates, proteins and micronutrients. The horse requires carbohydrates in the form of soluble sugars and starches. A horse's digestive system can cope with certain fats as well, even though these are not natural foods. Fats may be a useful energy source when a horse is in strong work and requires a higher energy diet than it might otherwise be possible to consume in a day.

Protein in a diet is much misunderstood by horse owners. Proteins are building blocks, not energy sources. Growing animals require relatively high levels of good quality protein and sick and pregnant animals have increased protein requirements. Horses in work do not. They only require sufficient protein to replace any muscle proteins broken down by exercise. Cellulose fibre in grass and hay is changed to usable nutrients by bacteria in the horse's large colon. If too much protein is fed, it will be broken down to provide energy but this is a very inefficient and costly way to produce energy.

The horse can manufacture or obtain all its vitamin requirements when out to grass. Only in exceptional circumstances are vitamin supplements required. Mineral levels can pose a problem because the level of one may interfere with the absorbtion of another. Commercial feeds are balanced for such problems. Home-mixed feeds are not. Adding extra ingredients to a commercially balanced feed may completely upset the vitamin/mineral balance.

It is not within the scope of a book such as this to provide sample diets for different classes of horse. Apart from anything else, the nutritional value of ingredients such as oats or hay varies tremendously from sample to sample. For all but the most experienced horsemaster it is advisable to stick to manufactured foods from a reputable supplier. One point must be made however, and that is that oats are not God's gift to horses. They form no part of their 'natural' diet. Their traditional success as a horse feed is based on their low energy content in relation to the volume of food rather than anything else. They do not provide a balanced diet on their own, and their addition to a balanced mix will promptly unbalance it.

Disease prevention

The best way to avoid digestive problems is to provide a constant, unchanging supply of food. Any change in diet can result in fibre not being digested because the particular blend of bacteria required to digest it is not present. An impaction may be the result, even where the change is from a concentrate to a grass diet. More nutrients will always be absorbed from several small meals than from one large one, and these meals should be evenly spaced out and their timing kept constant.

There are a number of conditions, notably laminitis (see page 76) and azoturia (see page 155), where overfeeding plays a role. The horse owner's standard reaction to a lack of performance is to feed more high-energy food. This is the opposite of what is usually required. It is perhaps worth noting that there is no such thing as a 'heating' food; the lively behaviour put down to feeding such substances is just the result of a relatively high carbohydrate diet. All feedstuffs have a different concentration of accessible energy per unit weight, and a different weight per unit volume. A scoop of one does not contain the same amount of energy as a scoop of another, nor does it weigh the same.

Feeding must be precisely related to the work being done. Anything which results in work being reduced must be accompanied immediately by a reduction of feeding levels. It is always safer for increases in food to lag behind any weight loss resulting from increased work. In other words, we should wait until we have proof (in the form of a slight weight loss) that a horse needs extra food before increasing the ration. If we increase the ration when the horse could actually have coped without an increase we may trigger azoturia.

Horse owners should make sure that they are familiar with common poisonous plants. It is too late to look up what ragwort looks like, for example (see page 78), when a horse is already showing signs of poisoning. Poisonous plants pose more of a risk when there is little grass available due to over-grazing or seasonal factors. Some plants, such as ragwort, can also be poisonous in hay so it is worth keeping an eye open when filling hay nets as well.

Regular deworming may prevent sufficient build-up of intestinal worms to cause clinical symptoms, but it does not prevent there being any worms at all. As worms are spread in faeces, the higher the concentration of faeces on a paddock, the higher the risk of worms. A high density of horses per unit area means a high risk of picking up worms. Over-grazing increases the risk of worms because it encourages horses to graze rough parts of the paddock which they normally reserve

DEWORMER	EXTRA ACTIVITY	PASTE AVAILABLE	RESISTANCE
DICHLORVOS	also treats bots	–	+
FEBANTEL		–	+
HALOXON	some bot activity	+	+
OXIBENDAZOLE		+	+
MEBENDAZOLE	needs higher dose for lungworm		+ +
THIABENDAZOLE	needs double dose for ascarids	+	+
FEBENDAZOLE	needs higher dose for lungworm & worm larvae	+	+
OXFENDAZOLE	some lungworm activity	+	+
IVERMECTIN	active lungworm & worm larvae	+	No resistance reported despite years of use
METRIPHONATE	only bots, ascarids & oxyuris	+	+
PYRANTEL	active tapeworms at double dose	+	No resistance reported despite years of use

Fig. 76 *A chart showing the different horse dewormers and their uses*

for dunging. Picking up and removing faeces regularly reduces the risk. Harrowing the paddock exposes the worm larvae and eggs to drying and temperature variations which kill them. Topping pasture reduces the risk of infection because worm larvae tend to crawl to the top of grass stalks where they will be most readily consumed.

Not all anthelmintics, or dewormers, kill the same species of worm at the normal dose rate. It is important to check by reading the manufacturer's literature that you are using the right drug for your expected problems, and at the right dosage. There is a gradual increase in the incidence of drug resistance in worms, especially the small strongyles *(Fig. 76)*. Unfortunately this resistance tends to extend to all drugs of the same family. Changing dewormers every time you deworm your horse is not a reliable way to avoid resistance developing. It is better to use a drug such as ivermectin or pyrantel, against which no resistance has yet developed. Then you do not need to change the drug except in special circumstances—for example, to control tapeworms or lungworm. Resistance is a particular problem in the benzamidazole group of dewormers, which includes many dewormers still widely sold. Deworming usually needs to be carried out every six to eight weeks if further contamination of the pasture is to be avoided.

Acorn poisoning

Symptoms The horse becomes very dull. Initially it is constipated, although eventually this may change to persistent diarrhoea due to the development of gastroenteritis. The kidneys are damaged, and the urine becomes dark in colour.

Cause Tannin in the acorns and leaves is the main toxic substance. Poisoning appears to be more common in some years than in others.

Treatment Large amounts of liquid paraffin, or mineral oil are given by stomach tube in order to speed up removal of the plant material.

Prognosis This depends on the amount of kidney damage. The kidney has poor powers of recovery.

Ascarid worms

Symptoms These worms usually affect only young horses because older animals develop immunity. The foal loses weight because of damage caused to the intestinal wall and occasionally due to the blockage of bile ducts. The worms may also obstruct the intestine. Migrating ascarids pass through the lungs, giving rise to coughing, a raised temperature and a nasal discharge *(Fig. 77)*.

Cause Parascaris equorum is picked up from the pasture by foals. The worm eggs which eventually pass out in the foal's faeces can lie dormant until the following year.

Treatment Most anthelmintics are effective against ascarids at normal doses. Treatment needs to be carried out every six to eight weeks to keep the foal clear.

Prognosis Good.

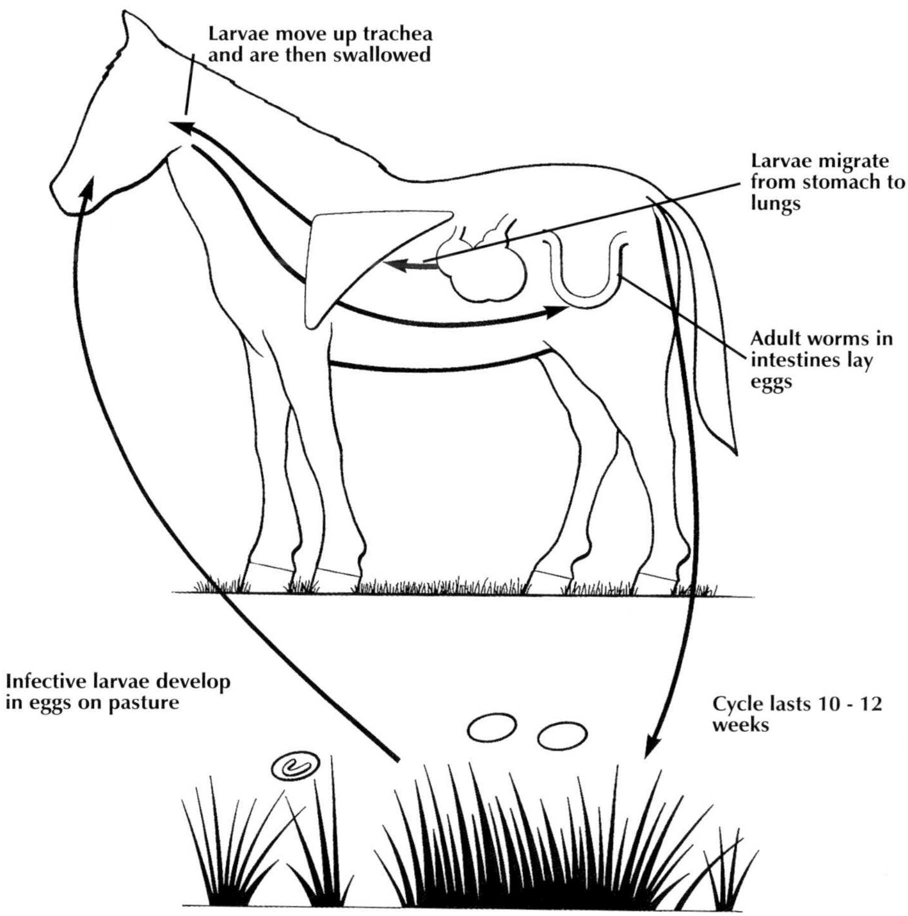

Fig. 77 *The life cycle of Parascaris equorum*

Bots

Symptoms The presence of large numbers of bot larvae in the stomach in winter can cause the horse to lose condition.

Cause The Gasterophilus fly lays its eggs on the horse's body, especially the legs, during the summer months (*Fig. 78*). The larvae are licked off the hair, passing through to the stomach, where they spend the winter before passing out in the faeces next spring (*Fig. 79*).

Treatment Most anthelmintics are ineffective against bots. Ivermectin and dichlorvos have good activity. Dosing is carried out between November and January.

Prognosis Good.

Choke

Symptoms A highly distressed horse will not eat or drink and has a sudden nasal discharge (*Fig. 80*). A swelling may be visible on the lower left side of the neck.

Cause A solid object, such as a large piece of carrot or potato, or a feedstuff such as dry sugar beet pulp or a hay cube swells rapidly after contact with saliva, until it lodges in and blocks the oesophagus (*Fig. 81*).

Treatment Muscle relaxants may reduce spasm of the muscles in the oesophageal wall, and allow the object to pass on. Accumulated saliva may be sucked out via a stomach tube, reducing its chance of entering the trachea (windpipe). Alternatively, introducing small quantities of water via a stomach tube and then removing it may gradually wash away impacted sugar beet pulp. Care must be taken to avoid causing permanent damage to the oesophageal wall, which might predispose to further impactions.

Prognosis Good if treatment is started early enough.

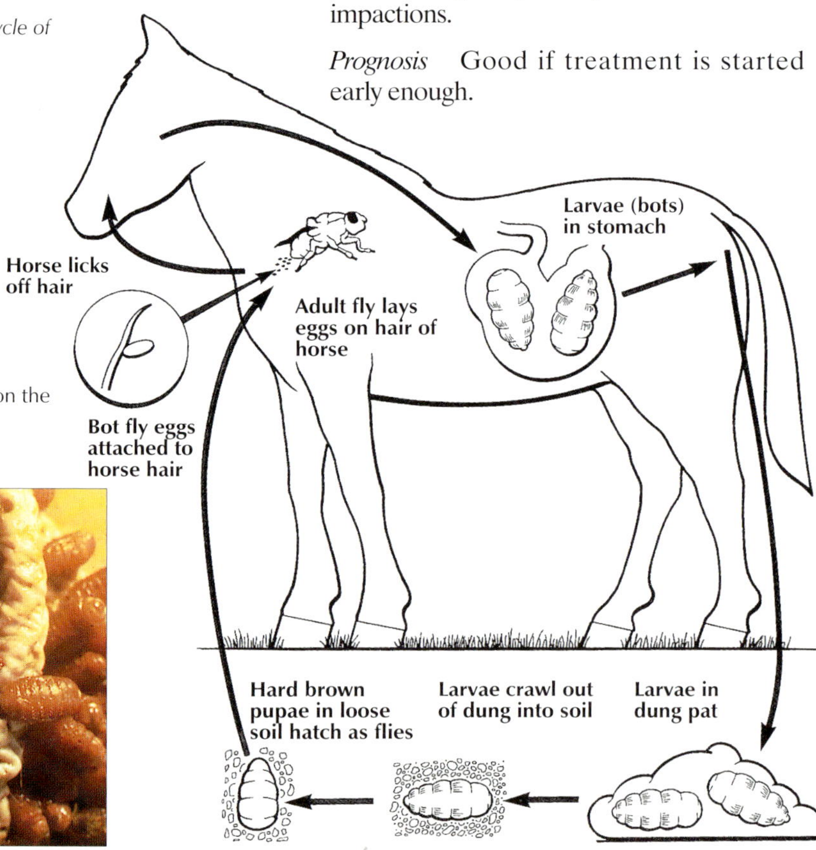

Fig. 78 *The life cycle of the horse bot fly*

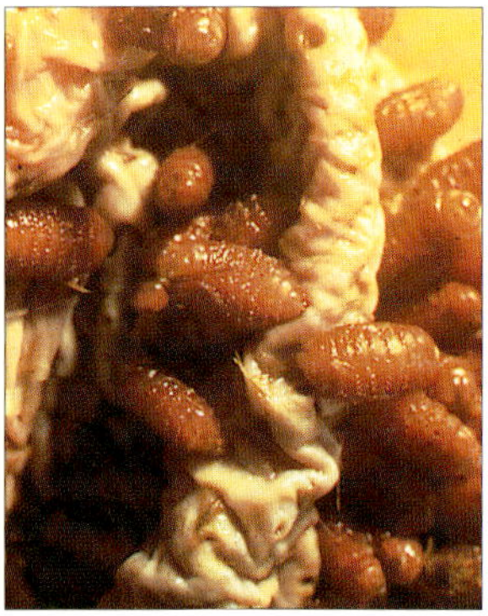

Fig. 79 Bot larvae on the lining of a horse's stomach.

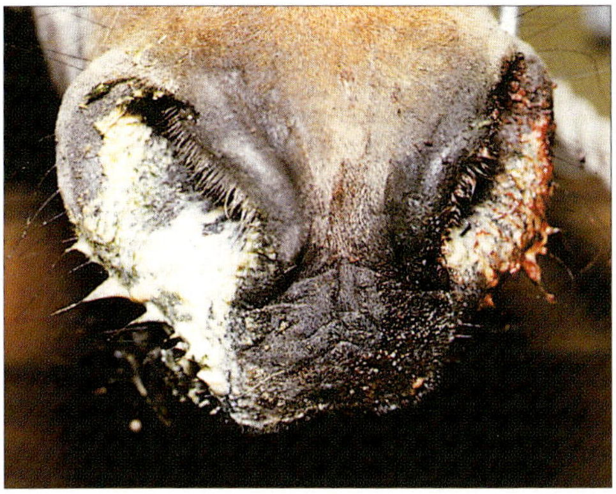

Fig. 80 Frothy nasal discharge of a horse with choke.

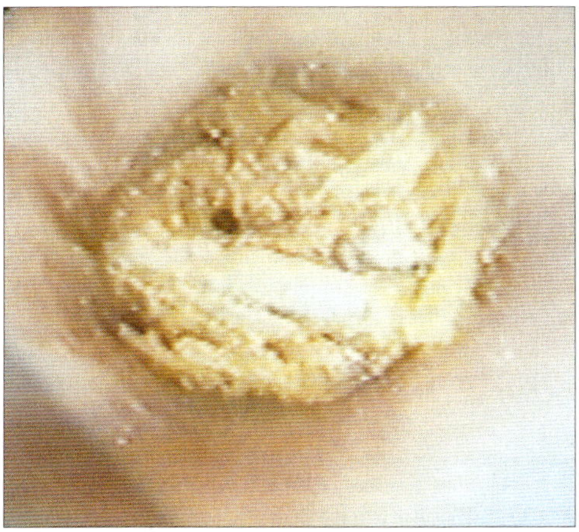

Fig. 81 Marked narrowing of the oesophagus of a horse which had an oesophageal stricture, a fibrous narrowing of the oesophagus due to repeated choke.

Chronic liver disease

Symptoms The first sign is usually a progressive loss of weight. The horse may lose its appetite. Eventually the horse may become sleepy, pressing its head against the wall and staggering aimlessly. Blood samples reveal that increased amounts of certain enzymes, such as sorbitol dehydrogenase, aspartate amino transferase and gamma glutamyl transpeptidase have been released by the damaged liver. Because the liver is involved in digestion, blood glucose levels are usually low. A liver biopsy will reveal the extent and nature of the damage.

Cause Tumours, toxic chemicals and plants, and fatty infiltration of the liver (usually in particularly fat animals) are the commonest causes of chronic liver disease.

Treatment A high-carbohydrate, low-protein diet is important. Glucose and B complex vitamins in particular should be supplemented.

Prognosis Because fibrosis and obstruction of the bile ducts is such a feature of chronic liver disease, the prognosis is poor.

Clostridal diarrhoea

Symptoms Sudden onset of profuse watery diarrhoea. Temperature may be raised. Dehydration and shock often occur. In acute cases death may occur within 24 hours.

Cause Intestinal proliferation of *Clostridium perfringens.*

Treatment "Sour milk" can produce a rapid improvement. Fluid therapy may be needed to reverse the dehydration.

Prognosis Guarded.

Colitis X

Symptoms Similar to those of acute salmonellosis (see page 79). The profuse water diarrhoea starts suddenly, and rapidly leads to dehydration and often death. Colic is severe *(See over page, Fig. 82).*

Cause No specific cause is known. There is usually a history of stress such as movement to new surroundings and/or worming or antibiotic administration. Shock may result from the changes; these can be detected by examining the lining of the caecum and large colon post mortem.

Treatment Fluid and electrolytes must be given to reverse the dehydration. Non-steroidal anti-inflammatory drugs help to control shock due to the absorption of endotoxins through the damaged bowel wall.

Prognosis The condition is often fatal.

Foal heat diarrhoea

Symptoms A profuse water diarrhoea in the foal, starting around 6 to 12 days after birth. It occurs at the same time as the mare has her first oestrus period after foaling.

Cause It used to be assumed that substances such as histamine are present in the milk which the foal drinks at this time, and that they cause the diarrhoea. Doubt has now been cast on this as the cause because even foals reared artificially away from the mare still develop diarrhoea at this time.

Treatment In the vast majority of cases no treatment is required, and the diarrhoea stops after 5 - 7 days. Antibiotics are not required unless there is definite evidence that a secondary infection has become established.

Prognosis Good.

Gastric ulceration

Symptoms Ulceration occurs most commonly in foals under four months of age. The foal is depressed and may have persistent diarrhoea. Occasionally this may be a cause of sudden death in very young foals. The ulcers may be seen with an endoscope in some foals. Pepsinogen levels in the blood tend to be high.

Cause Stress is an important factor in the condition, especially in foals which already have diarrhoea from other, usually infectious, causes.

Treatment Drugs used for the treatment of ulcers in man may be successful in foals. Fluid and electrolyte therapy may be indicated for the diarrhoea. Substances such as bismuth subcitrate given by mouth may provide a protective layer over the ulcer.

Prognosis Poor.

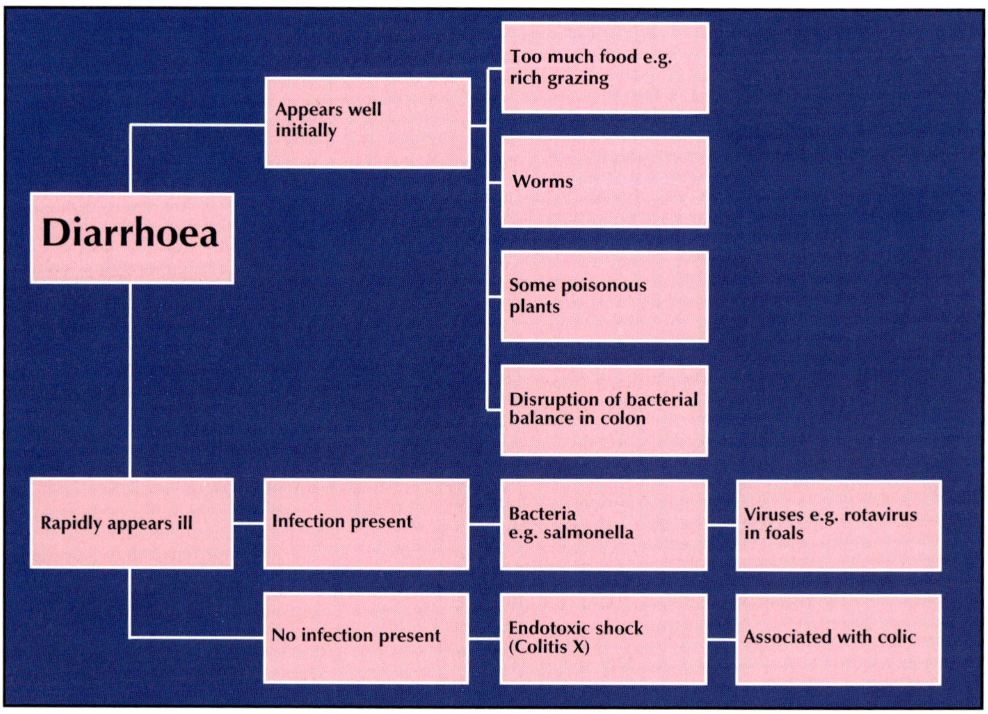

Fig. 82 *The causes of diarrhoea in the horse*

Grass sickness

Symptoms The condition may be acute with death occurring within 48 hours, but in chronic cases the horse deteriorates gradually over a number of weeks. In the latter the first symptom may be a loss of condition. Normal bowel movements cease, and their contents become dry and hard, while the stomach becomes distended with greenish fluid. The horse loses its ability to swallow, and may stand over food or water dribbling saliva. Twitching of the muscles, especially those over the shoulders, may be seen. Cases are more likely near the coast, shortly after some change in grazing management in the spring.

Cause The cause is thought to be toxic. So far all attempts to isolate the culprit have been unsuccessful. Grass sickness is basically a problem of the nervous system supplying the bowels, and characteristic changes may be seen in the nerves examined under the microscope after death. Multiple cases often occur on a premises over succeeding years.

Treatment
Treatment with the drug cisapride may maintain bowel contractions and so keep the horse alive until it can cure itself, but in many cases euthanasia is the only course open.

Prognosis Poor.

Hernia

Symptoms A soft swelling underneath the skin where a short length of intestines has escaped from the abdominal cavity. If the loop of intestines becomes pinched so that normal movement of contents is prevented, it will become hard and painful. The hernia is then said to be strangulated.

Cause Hernias most commonly occur where the umbilicus is attached in the foal (umbilical hernia) or in the groin of the male (inguinal hernia).

Treatment Small hernias may not require any treatment because it is considered that the risk of strangulation is very low. Larger hernias require surgery to replace the intestines and to close the hole in the abdominal wall.

Prognosis Good unless strangulation has already occurred.

Hyperlipaemia

Symptoms The horse is dull and not feeding or drinking. Blood samples show high levels of triglycerides (part of the fat molecule), and the blood may even look milky on standing because of the fat it contains.

Cause Stress increases energy requirements which are not met from glucose metabolism due to inadequate intake. Fat is mobilised into the bloodstream in an attempt to deal with the problem. Shetland ponies and donkeys are especially susceptible, and females more so than males.

Treatment Remove any stress. Ensure good level of glucose intake, initially by IV infusion and then by mouth. Insulin has been used to raise carbohydrate metabolism. Heparin has been used to remove fat from the blood but has the side-effect of reducing blood clotting.

Prognosis Poor once the condition is established.

Impactive colic

Symptoms Because the pain associated with an impaction is a steady chronic pain, the horse appears subdued. Often it will spend most of the time lying down, avoiding movement. It may continue to pass faeces for 24 to 36 hours after symptoms first appear. Indeed, there may be a history of slight diarrhoea temporarily. The colic may persist for several days with the horse becoming more and more distressed.

Cause Impactions are usually due to a failure to digest the fibrous part of the horse's diet, perhaps because the hay or other feed has been recently changed and the bacteria in the large colon have not adapted to the new fibre content. Dental disorders and lack of water predispose to impactions, as do intestinal parasites. The various changes which take place in the diameter and direction of the alimentary tract encourage the build-up of fibrous faeces. Once established, more fluid is absorbed out of the impacted material, and more material collects behind the impaction.

Treatment Drugs such as liquid paraffin or mineral oil, need to be given in large quantities via a stomach tube. Because of disturbances to the balance of the body fluids, intravenous fluid therapy may be necessary. In some cases surgery may be indicated.

Prognosis The prognosis is guarded. If marked shock and fluid imbalances occur the outlook may be poor.

Laminitis

Symptoms The classic symptom of laminitis—inflammation of the sensitive laminae between the pedal bone and the hoof—is heat in the hoof of one or more feet (see also page 151). It is quite possible, however, to have laminitis without any apparent heat. There is often a marked pulse along the artery leading to the foot as it passes down the pastern. The horse is lame, but the severity of the pain is masked by the fact that all four feet may be affected. In chronic cases the hoof becomes distorted, and the alteration in the angle of the pedal bone may result in it pressing through the sole of the foot *(Fig. 83)*.

Cause Although toxic shock, especially in mares after foaling, and some generalised infections can trigger off laminitis, the commonest cause is a high carbohydrate diet (including rich pasture). Endotoxins from the gut result in blood shunting around the coronet rather than supplying the laminae. Degeneration and tearing of the laminae may allow rotation of the pedal bone due to unopposed tension from the flexor tendon.

Treatment The triggering factor must first be rectified, for example by taking the affected animal off its lush pasture. It is vitally important that the foot is trimmed in order to maintain the correct angle between the pedal bone and the ground, even if this requires radical removal of horn. A heart bar shoe may then help in chronic cases. Frog pads may be used if the horse is not shod. Pain-killing drugs may be necessary, and drugs which dilate the affected blood vessels are also useful. Acetylpromazine reduces blood pressure to allow fuller foot circulation.

Prognosis Some animals are particularly susceptible to laminitis, and have repeated attacks if the level of carbohydrate in their diet changes at all. Even chronic cases can often be returned to normal if sufficient attention is paid to the trimming of their feet etc.

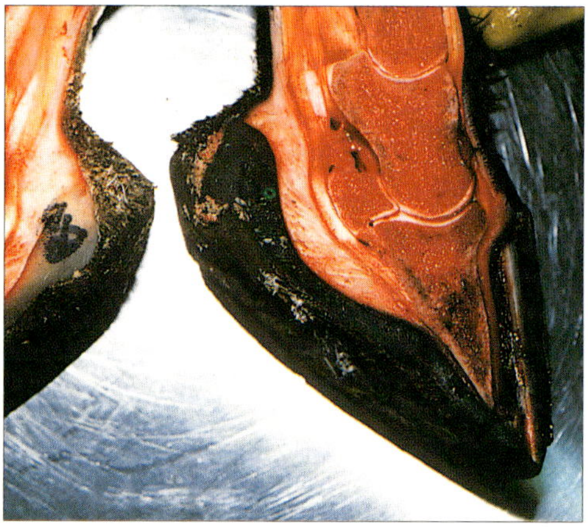

Fig. 83 *A cross-section through a horse's foot – a post mortem specimen.* The pedal bone has rotated.

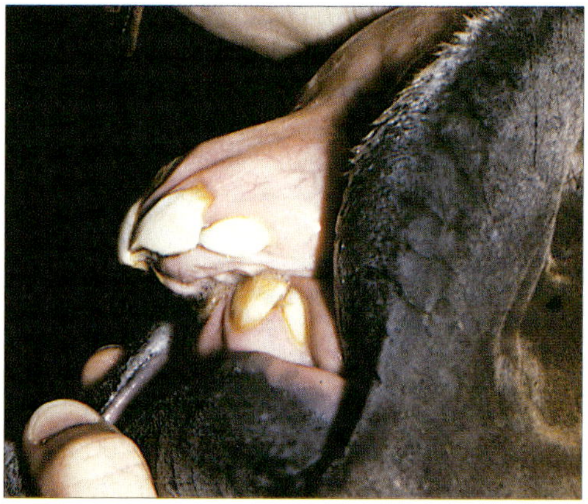

Fig. 84 *Parrot mouth*
The upper jaw fails to bite with the lower jaw.

Lead poisoning

Symptoms Symptoms usually develop slowly as the lead accumulates in the body. Diarrhoea and mild colic are followed by stiffness and difficulty in moving. The horse loses weight. Swallowing may become difficult. A whistling noise is often heard as the horse breathes in, due to paralysis of the nerve supplying the laryngeal muscles.

Cause Pasture near busy roads can become contaminated with lead from petrol fumes. Lead pipes in the water supply and lead paint are common sources.

Treatment A high phosphorus diet stimulates transfer of the lead to the bones, where it is inactive. Calcium disodium EDTA increases excretion of the lead from the body.

Prognosis The prognosis is guarded because the symptoms may be well developed before the cause is diagnosed.

Parrot mouth

Symptoms The upper incisor teeth project in front of the lower incisors *(Fig. 84)*. They may not make any contact with the lower incisors. Such horses fail to thrive at pasture because they cannot graze properly. Partial contact between the jaws can give unusual wear on the teeth, and so foil any attempt to age the horse by its teeth.

Cause It is a congenital fault which may improve as the foal grows, but will not change once development is complete.

Treatment No treatment is possible. Affected horses require permanent supplementary feed.

Prognosis It is suggested that affected horses should not be used for breeding.

Pin worm

Symptoms Affected horses rub their tails, causing hair loss.

Cause The female *Oxyuris equi* worm lives just inside the anus, coming out on to the skin to lay its eggs and thus causing the irritation *(Fig. 85)*.

Treatment Many anthelmintics are effective against *Oxyuris.*

Prognosis Good.

Fig.85 *The life cycle of Oxyuris equi – the pin worm*

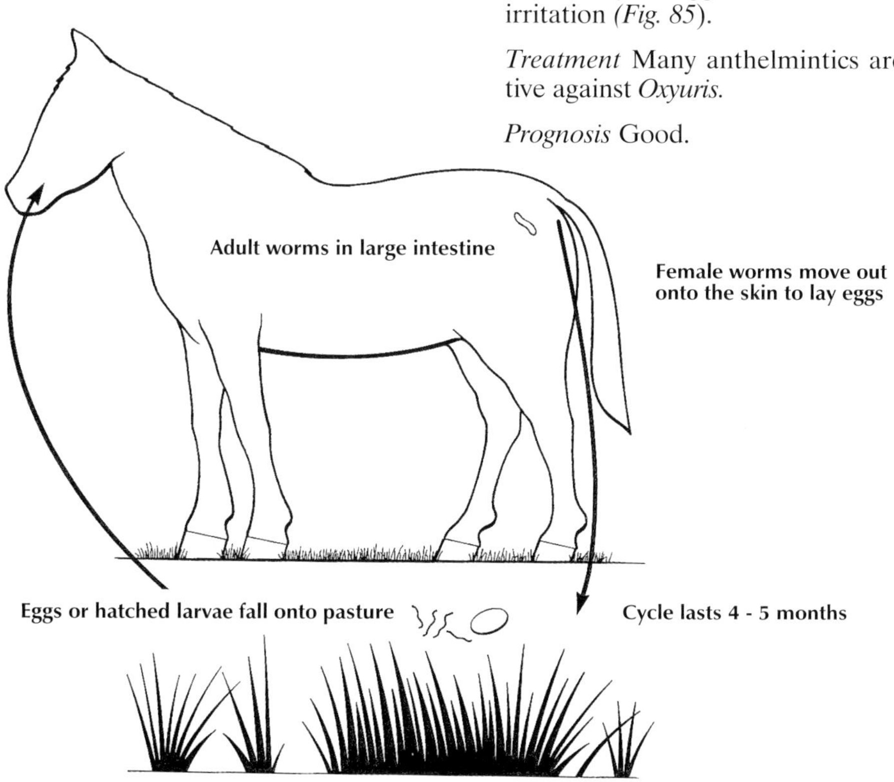

Protein-losing enteropathy

Symptoms The horse loses weight, in some cases very rapidly. It may develop oedema of the lower limbs and ventral abdomen. It is lethargic. Initially, the horse's appetite is not affected. Protein levels in the blood are markedly reduced.

Cause Any disease which damages a significant length of the bowel can be a cause as proteins are no longer absorbed. The oedema is caused by insufficient protein in the blood to hold water inside the blood vessels rather than out in the general tissues. A lymphosarcoma tumour of the intestinal wall is one of the most common causes. Severe worm damage to the intestines may also cause the condition.

Treatment No treatment is possible.

Prognosis Guarded. If the plasma protein level drops below 20g per litre the prognosis is poor.

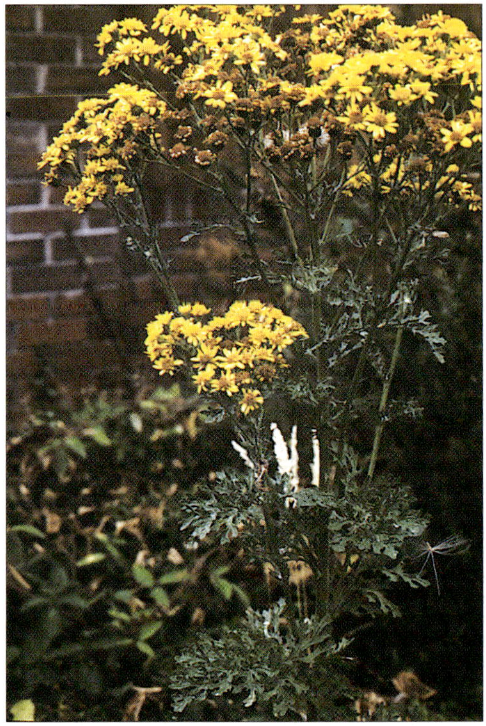

Fig. 86 *A ragwort flower*

Ragwort poisoning

Symptoms Usually appear after chronic poisoning over a period of time. A slow loss of weight may take some time to become obvious. The horse's appetite may also gradually decrease over a period of a month or more. Because the liver is damaged, any of the symptoms of liver disease may occur, and this helps diagnosis because a blood sample shows raised levels of the enzymes normally associated with the liver. Affected horses may be very depressed and hang their heads down. Because this may also be associated with a rather staggering walk, the disease is sometimes called 'sleepy staggers'.

Cause Ragwort *(Fig. 86)* and most other members of the Senecio family of plants, including common groundsel and stinking willie weed, are poisonous to the horse. The living plant is bitter, so the horse only eats it when other food is short *(Fig. 87)*. Unfortunately, even dried ragwort in hay is poisonous. It is said that a horse needs to eat over 20 kilos (45 lbs) of the plant to cause symptoms to appear unless the poison is consumed over a very short time.

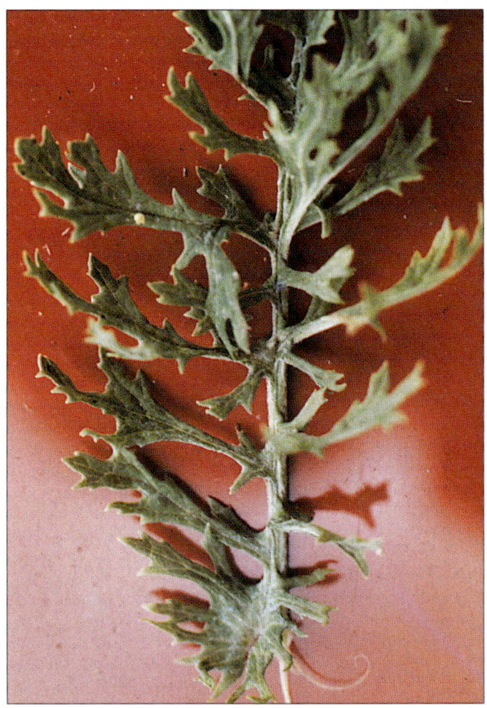

Fig. 87 *The ragwort plant*

Treatment There is no specific treatment for ragwort poisoning, although intravenous dextrose or oral glucose may help the liver function. The best way to avoid the problem is by not allowing the horse to graze in, or make hay from, contaminated fields. The only sure way to remove the plant from a paddock is by literally pulling it up by its roots.

Prognosis Most affected horses die.

Retained meconium

Symptoms This is a condition affecting foals during the first four or five days of life. Initially the foal may stop suckling the mare. It might be seen standing with its tail raised up in the air, possibly even straining to pass some faeces, but without any success. As the condition progresses, the foal may show a raised temperature. It may even show typical colic symptoms, rolling on the ground or kicking at its abdomen.

Cause The cause is a failure to pass the meconium, the faeces which have accumulated in the posterior part of the foal's large intestine while it was developing inside the mare. Such meconium is hard in consistency and a dark, sometimes greenish-black, colour. It may occupy 46 - 60cm (18 - 24in) of the bowels at birth. Because colt foals have a narrower passage through the bony pelvis than filly foals, they are much more susceptible to the condition. Most of the pain is caused by the fact that the normal peristaltic waves of contraction and retraction, which pass along the bowels after the foal has suckled milk come to a 'dead end' at the impaction.

Treatment Small quantities of meconium can be removed by hand as long as great care is taken not to damage the rectal wall. Fluid enemas using soap and water or liquid paraffin will soften the pellets and hopefully stimulate the bowel wall contractions by expanding the walls. Great care must be taken not to damage the rectum when inserting the tube for the enema, and only small quantities of fluid should be given. Micro-enemas consisting of sodium atrate, sodium alkylsulphoacetate and sorbic acid are particularly useful because they avoid such damage and are safe and effective to use. Treatment must be continued until all the meconium has been passed. The only way to be sure of this is to have seen the foal pass normal soft orange/yellow faeces. The symptoms disappear very rapidly once all the meconium has been passed.

Prognosis Good with treatment. In unskilful hands the treatment may cause more lasting damage than the condition itself.

Salmonellosis

Symptoms Painful acute diarrhoea with a raised body temperature are the usual symptoms. Many horses exposed to the infection become carriers, possibly becoming ill at a later date. Stress such as pregnancy, transportation, surgery and antibiotic therapy can trigger the disease.

Cause Infection may be airborne, via contaminated feed, or by general environmental contamination. Salmonella are a large family of bacteria. It is necessary to culture the particular bacterium responsible from the faeces or from internal organs such as the liver to confirm the diagnosis. Repeated sampling may be necessary before this is successful.

Treatment

Replacement of the fluid and salts lost in the diarrhoea is more important than the killing of the infectious organism itself. Antibiotics should only be used when laboratory tests show that the particular strain isolated is sensitive to the proposed drug.

Prognosis If fluid and salt balances can be maintained (sometimes a difficult and expensive task) the prognosis is fair.

Selenium poisoning

Symptoms In its acute form selenium poisoning can cause nervous symptoms and death. More commonly in 'chronic alkali disease' there is a marked decrease in horn quality, often associated with laminitis. There may be hair-loss from the mane and tail.

Cause In some areas the soil has high levels of selenium, which are reflected in the levels in grass, hay and cereals grown on them. Accidental feed contamination has occurred.

Treatment Only symptomatic treatment is possible.

Prognosis
In acute cases the prognosis is fair as long as the source is removed. In chronic cases the prognosis is guarded as horses developing laminitis may need to be put down on humane grounds.

Small strongyles
Symptoms The presence of large numbers of these worms can cause unthriftiness and diarrhoea. Symptoms are most commonly seen in the first five months of the year in the northern hemisphere. Many species suck blood from the bowel wall.

Cause There are several species of small worms, grouped together as the Cyanthostomes, which cause no problem unless present in large numbers *(Fig. 88)*.

Treatment
Drug resistance is worse for these worms than for any other. Pyrantel or ivermectin should be used in preference to any other drugs because no resistance has yet been discovered to these two drugs. The short life-cycle of the worms means that new infestations constantly occur, so treatment is necessary every six to eight weeks.

Prognosis Good.

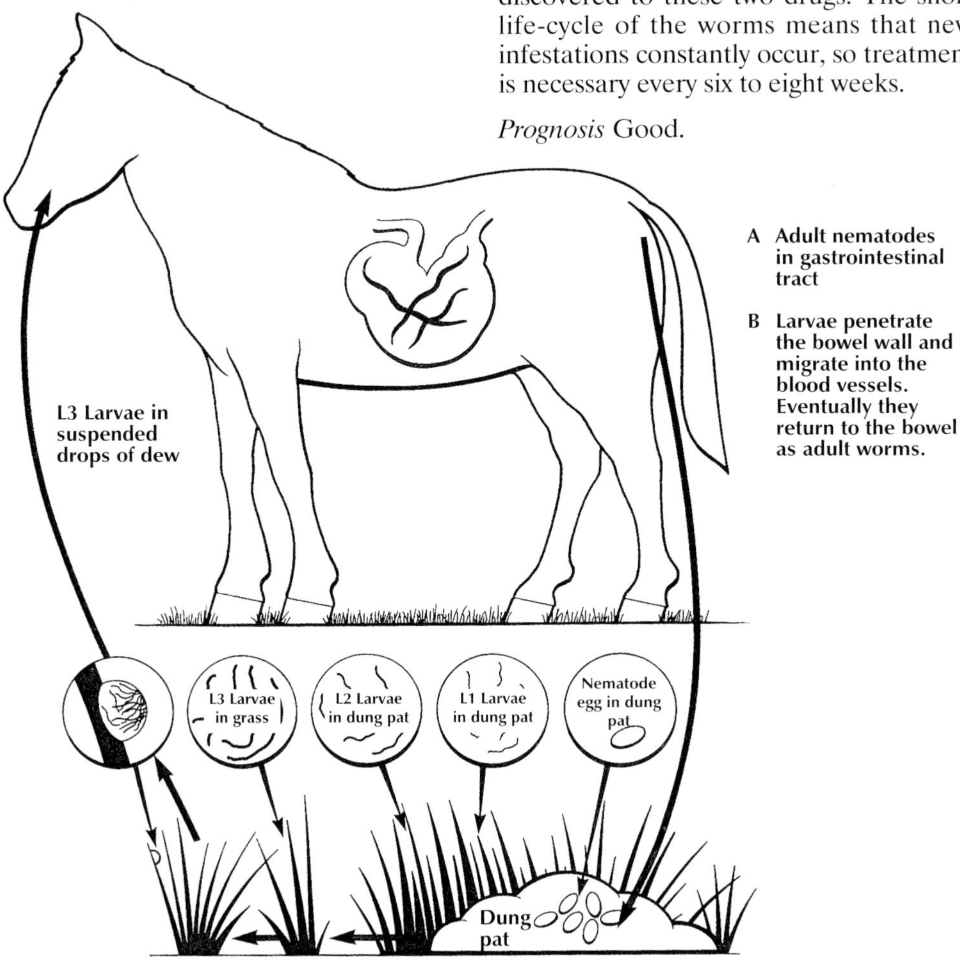

Fig. 88 The life cycle of the small strongyle worms (A) and strongylus vulgaris (B).

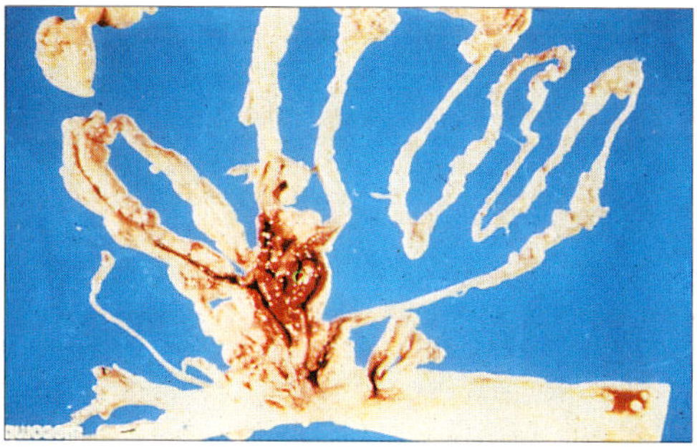

Fig. 89 Disruption of the blood supply to a horse's intestines as a result of damage from migrating Strongylus larvae – post mortem specimen.

Spasmodic colic

Symptoms As its name implies, the horse has occasional bouts of colic lasting perhaps 30 minutes, during which the pain may be quite acute, interspersed with periods of apparent normality.

Cause There can be many causes, and it may not be possible to arrive at a precise cause. Even nervous excitement from a 'fright' can trigger the colic.

Treatment Because the pain can trigger spasm of the muscles in the bowel wall, which causes further pain, analgesics should be given to relieve it, break the cycle and so relieve the condition. Drugs which relax the smooth muscles in the bowel wall, such as hyoscine, also help to relieve the muscle spasm. Constant walking around of the horse is not necessary and does not prevent the affected bowels from becoming twisted upon themselves (see twisted bowel, page 83).

Prognosis As long as there is no serious physical cause for the colic, the prognosis with treatment is good.

Strongylus vulgaris

Symptoms The adult worm sucks blood from the bowel wall, and in large numbers it can cause anaemia. During their development the worm larvae migrate to the blood vessels which supply the loops of the intestines and stay there for several months. They thus interfere with the blood supply to the intestines *(Fig. 89)*. This can cause a loss of condition due to reduced bowel function. It can also cause colic ranging from mild recurring bouts to an acute colic.

Cause Strongylus vulgaris larvae are ingested during grazing *(Fig. 88)*. They have a long life-cycle and it can be up to six months before they have matured to egg-laying adult worms back in the intestine.

Treatment Most anthelmintics are usually effective against adult *strongylus vulgaris* but resistant strains of the worm can occur. This resistance will also apply to other drugs of the same family, for instance to all members of the group of compounds ending in -ndazole. Pyrantel and ivermectin have no resistance. Ivermectin alone has high efficacy against migrating strongyle larvae.

Prognosis Good

Tapeworms

Symptoms There are a number of cases where tapeworms have triggered off intestinal impactions. Tapeworms are certainly more common in horses than was at first thought.

Cause Anoplocephela is the most common species of tapeworm in the horse *(Fig. 90)*.

Treatment Pyrantel is effective at twice the normal dose.

Prognosis Good.

Tooth abscesses

Symptoms A painful swelling occurs around the infected tooth root. This can be readily seen on the lower jaw, but may be invisible in the upper jaw, where the roots of the molar teeth project into the nasal sinuses. As the abscess ruptures, pus drains either through a hole in the skin (the lower jaw) or down the nostril on the affected side (the upper jaw). The damaged tooth can be detected on X-ray.

Cause There is usually a history of some physical injury to the area around the tooth root, although it may be some time before the infection becomes apparent.

Treatment Antibiotics help control the infection, but the tooth usually needs to be removed. This removes the focus of infection and allows drainage of the pus.

Prognosis Recovery is good. Regular rasping of the molar teeth may be necessary to prevent the opposing tooth growing excessively long when no longer being worn down.

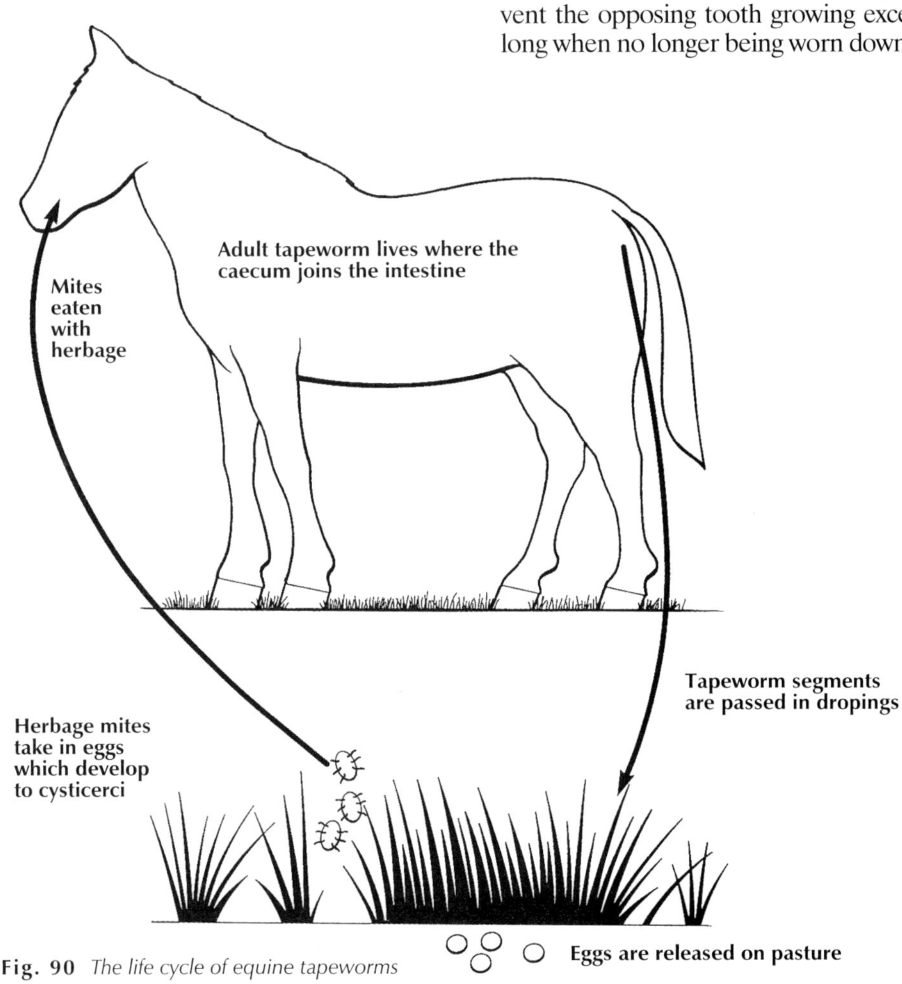

Fig. 90 *The life cycle of equine tapeworms*

Tooth problems

Symptoms The horse may not respond as well to the bit as the rider expects, and may throw its head around. Pain associated with chewing may result if the horse allows partially chewed food to drop out of its mouth ('quidding'). It may also reduce the amount of food consumed. Improper chewing of the food can result in colic as the rest of the alimentary tract fails to cope with the material passing along it. Affected horses may lose weight.

Cause The fact that the grinding surfaces of the molar teeth are set at an angle to the horizontal, coupled with the fact that the upper molars are wider than the lower molars, results in sharp points being formed on the outside edges of the upper molars and the inside edges of the lower molars. These sharp points rub against the tongue and the cheeks.

Treatment Rasping (or floating) the molar teeth files off the sharp edges and so removes the discomfort.

Prognosis Good.

Twisted and displaced bowel

Symptoms The horse shows severe signs of colic, with little or no remission. Analgesic drugs may have only limited effect on the pain. The membranes around the eye become brick-red and the pulse rate is very high. There is a steady deterioration in the horse's condition.

Cause There are a variety of ways in which parts of the digestive tract can twist on themselves, or become displaced within the abdomen. Similar symptoms occur when a short length of bowel starts to degenerate because of an obstruction to its blood supply. Worm damage to the blood vessels supplying the loops of bowel is a common cause of such an obstruction.

Treatment If physical displacement has occurred, or if the bowel wall has become necrotic (dead), surgery is the only treatment. Fluid therapy is a vital part of the treatment because of the shock associated with the bowel damage.

Prognosis Poor whenever colic surgery is required. The success rate is markedly increased by resorting to surgery earlier rather than later. It is also higher when performed by certain specialised units which can justify the high labour and drug costs.

Tyzzer's disease

Symptoms Sudden death may be the only symptom of this condition, which occurs in foals up to six weeks of age. Clinically affected foals have a high heart rate and jaundice. The liver becomes very swollen.

Cause The bacterium *Bacillus piliformis*.

Treatment Broad spectrum antibiotics are given, initially intravenously because of the rapid course of the disease.

Prognosis Poor unless the disease is mild enough to allow it to be diagnosed and treated before fatal liver damage has occurred.

Vitamin deficiencies

Symptoms Vitamin deficiency is rare in horses, and very rare indeed in horses which have any access to pasture. Lack of performance may be due to lack of thiamine (Vitamin B1) but never to lack of Vitamin B12. Lack of folic acid can cause anaemia, while low levels of Vitamin A or C may reduce resistance to disease.

Cause Vitamin deficiences are only likely to occur in horses under stress which have not had regular access to grass or good hay. Many vitamins which we can only obtain from our food are readily manufactured by the horse in its own body.

Treatment Vitamin supplements must always be fresh as they may deteriorate with incorrect storage. Many proprietary vitamin supplements have levels which are too low to be of value in a deficiency.

Prognosis Increasing vitamin levels completely reverses the symptoms in most cases.

Wolf teeth

Symptoms Resentment of pressure from the bit results in reduced performance, especially in flat work.

Cause Wolf teeth are small premolar teeth *(Fig. 91)*. They are only embedded in the gums, not into the bone, and so can 'rock' when the bit presses against them. Wolf teeth are not present in all horses. They are more common in the upper jaw than the lower one.

Treatment Removal of wolf teeth is relatively simple.

Prognosis Good.

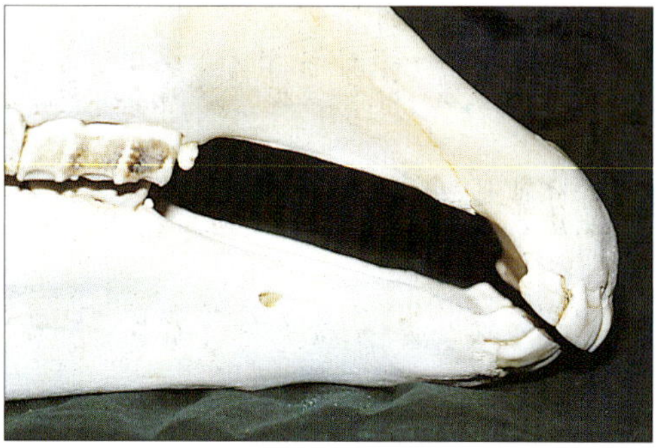

Fig. 91 Side view of a horse's skull showing a wolf tooth present in front of the larger molars.

Yew tree poisoning

Symptoms Sudden death is the usual symptom, with yew tree leaves being found in the mouth or stomach.

Cause The leaves and twigs are poisonous, although the berries are not *(Fig. 92)*.

Treatment There is no antidote.

Prognosis Affected horses always die.

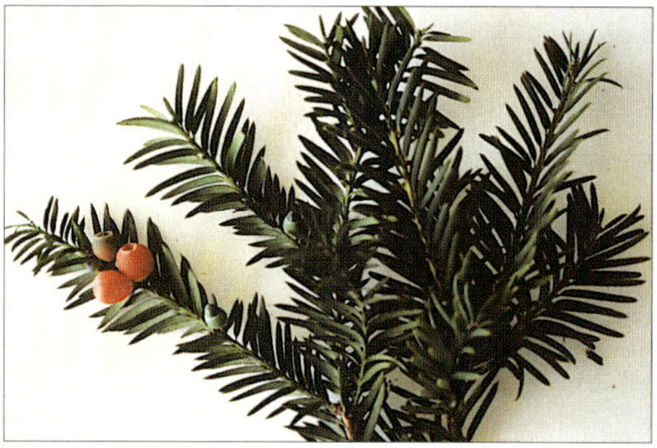

Fig. 92 *Yew leaves*

7: Horse breeding and the effect of reproductive problems

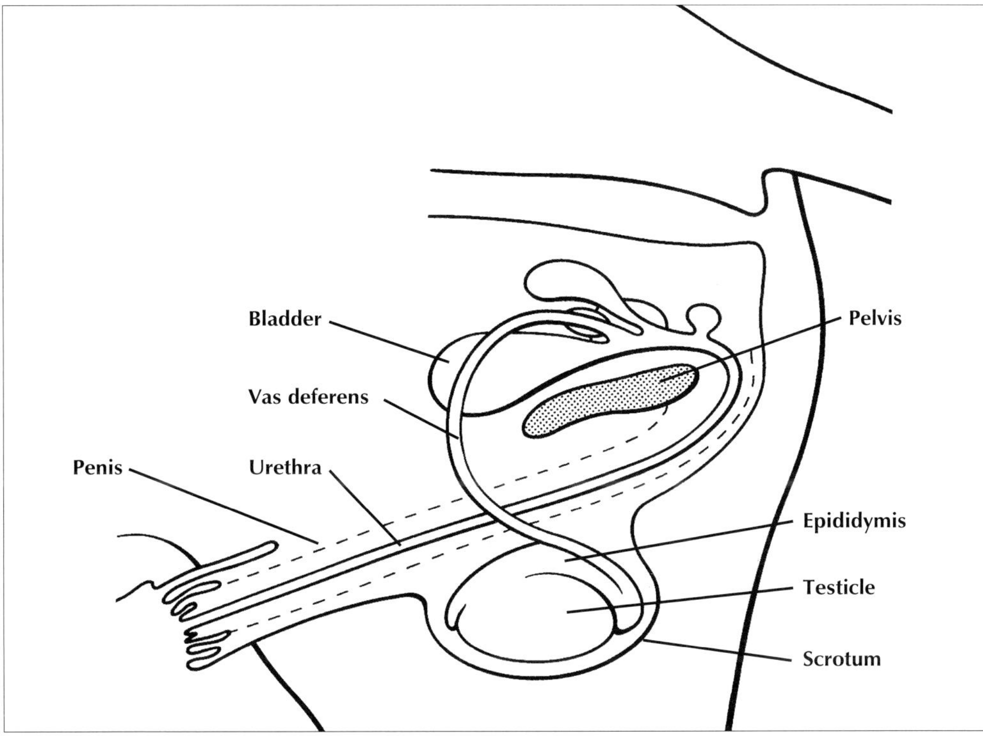

Fig. 93 *The stallion's reproductive system*

The male reproductive system

The male reproductive organ is the penis *(Fig. 93)*. For much of the time this is held inside a tunnel under the skin of the ventral abdomen which is known as the prepuce, or sheath. When the horse is relaxed its penis can hang down loosely under the body for at least twelve inches. Sedation produces the same effect.

This is obviously a very different organ to that which is so rigid when mating a mare. The difference lies in the amount of blood in the body of the penis. Within the penis is a sponge-like tissue called the corpus cavernosum. When blood flow out of the corpus cavernosum is restricted, it becomes full of blood under such pressure that it holds the penis erect. When, as a result of hormonal control, the blood is allowed to move out of the penis freely again, the penis collapses.

Apart from the corpus cavernosum, the other main structure of the penis is the urethra. This is the tube which links the bladder with the outside world, emptying at the tip of the penis. During the act of mating, however, the urethra carries semen from the sex organs. The surface of the penis is covered with specially adapted skin continuous with that lining the sheath. When the penis is retracted, this skin is folded up inside the sheath. When the penis is erect, it pulls the skin out rather like opening a concertina. There is a retractor muscle which pulls the penis back inside the sheath when it is not erect. The surface often has large quantities of a waxy substance called smegma, produced by glands in the skin. At the tip of the penis is an enlargement called the glans penis, where the urethra ends.

The most important sex glands are the two testicles. The left testicle is often larger than the right one. They pull down a sack of fine skin around them which is known as the scrotum. It is thought that having the testicles relatively exposed in this way helps to control their temperature, which needs to be slightly below that of the horse's normal internal body temperature. Inflammation of the testicle or the scrotum causes a rise in temperature, and can result in infertility. The testicles and scrotum lie between the back legs, and so are largely hidden from view.

The testicle itself consists of numerous compartments separated by partitions of connective tissue. Each of these compartments contains a tube called a seminiferous tubule. Sperm are produced along the length of these tubules, which join together at one end and drain in to the epididymis, a storage organ for the sperm. It extends over the top of the testicle, and finally empties into another tube called the vas deferens, which leads to the urethra.

The surgical cutting and/or tying off of the vas deferens prevents any sperm being released during mating, even though the stallion is in every other way an entire male. Such an operation is called a vasectomy, and is occasionally used to produce a 'teaser' stallion, which can tell whether the mares are in season and receptive to a stallion, without there being any risk of the teaser siring any foals himself. The vas deferens does not go by the direct subcutaneous route from the testicle to the penis. It passes into the abdomen and then out again to the urethra.

The vas deferens, a large artery and a vein which supply the testicle, and a muscle called the cremaster muscle (which can pull the testicle tight up against the body wall for protection or warmth) all make up the spermatic cord. This passes in through an opening in the abdominal wall which is known as the inguinal canal. The vas deferens finally empties into the urethra near to its emergence from the bladder. In this region there are also accessory sex glands which provide some of the fluid which dilutes the sperm and produce semen.

When a male foal is born, both testicles are usually already present in the scrotum, surrounded by a sheet of peritoneum (the membrane which lines the abdominal cavity). This is because they were originally formed inside the abdomen, near to the kidneys, but were pulled outside to the scrotum. Sometimes one or both of the testicles can move in and out of the inguinal canal during the first weeks or months of life. Many foals, therefore, do not appear to have any testicles, or appear to only have one present in the scrotum. The right testicle is often slightly larger than the one on the left. Occasionally intestines may also be present in the scrotum, giving a scrotal hernia *(Fig. 94)*.

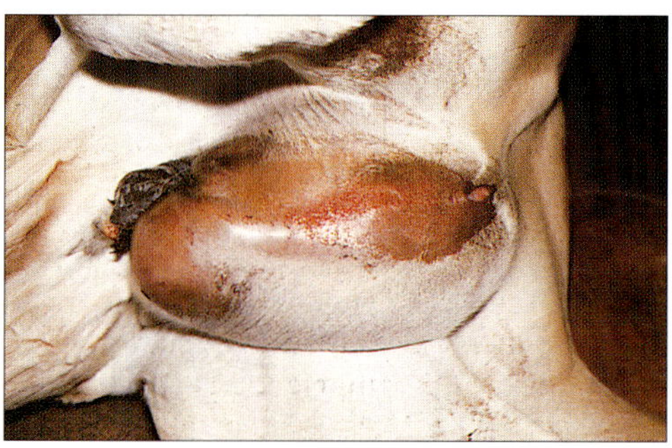

Fig. 94 *A scrotal hernia*

The testicles are also responsible for manufacturing the male hormone, testosterone. This is responsible for most of the male sexual characteristics, such as the desire to mate females, erection of the penis when aroused, and the aggression which a stallion needs in the wild. Removal of the testicles (castration), therefore removes both the desire to mate and the sperm that are needed for a successful mating. Opinions differ over when is the best time to castrate a male horse which is not wanted for breeding. The operation can be carried out at any age when the foal has become sexually mature (usually around six months of age). Stallions develop a 'crest' along the top of their neck, and some people feel that the muscles of the neck will not develop properly if the animal is castrated too early. All the evidence, however, points to there being little if any long-term advantage in leaving a male entire merely in the hope that it will help his physical development.

Young colts will naturally start mounting other horses, male or female, very early in their life. They may even attempt to mate their mothers. Their natural desire to prove their dominance also makes them less amenable to discipline than, say, mares. As a result, entire stallions which are not definitely needed for breeding are often neutered by castration. The resulting geldings take on more of the characteristics of mares in that they are less possessive and more amenable to control by man.

At castration a skin cut is made over each of the testicles in the scrotum. The testicles are brought outside the body and the spermatic cord is severed. To stop bleeding from the blood vessels the cord is either crushed or tied off with a ligature. The skin wounds are not usually closed by stitching because fluid tends to accumulate around the castration site, and it is important for this to be able to drain away rather than remain and possibly become infected. It is important that horses receive regular exercise during the week or two after castration in order to stimulate the circulation to remove any tissue fluid which accumulates. It is not sufficient just to hope that a horse standing in a field will move around enough to achieve the same result. It is also important that flies do not lay their eggs around the castration wound, where they can hatch out into maggots. This is why horses are not usually castrated during the heat of the summer. Nor are they castrated during frosty winter weather, when freezing may damage the tissues exposed in the scrotum.

Each millilitre of stallion semen can contain between 50 to 100 million sperm. As a stallion may ejaculate 40 to 80 millilitres at each mating, he is obviously providing an enormous number of sperm, only one of which will actually join with the mare's egg. Sperm look like tadpoles when examined under a microscope, and after mating swim up the mare's reproductive tract in search of a fertile egg. When potential stallions are being considered for breeding, much importance may be placed on the density of the sperm in the semen, the numbers of physically abnormal sperm present, and the amount of movement shown by the sperm as they move around.

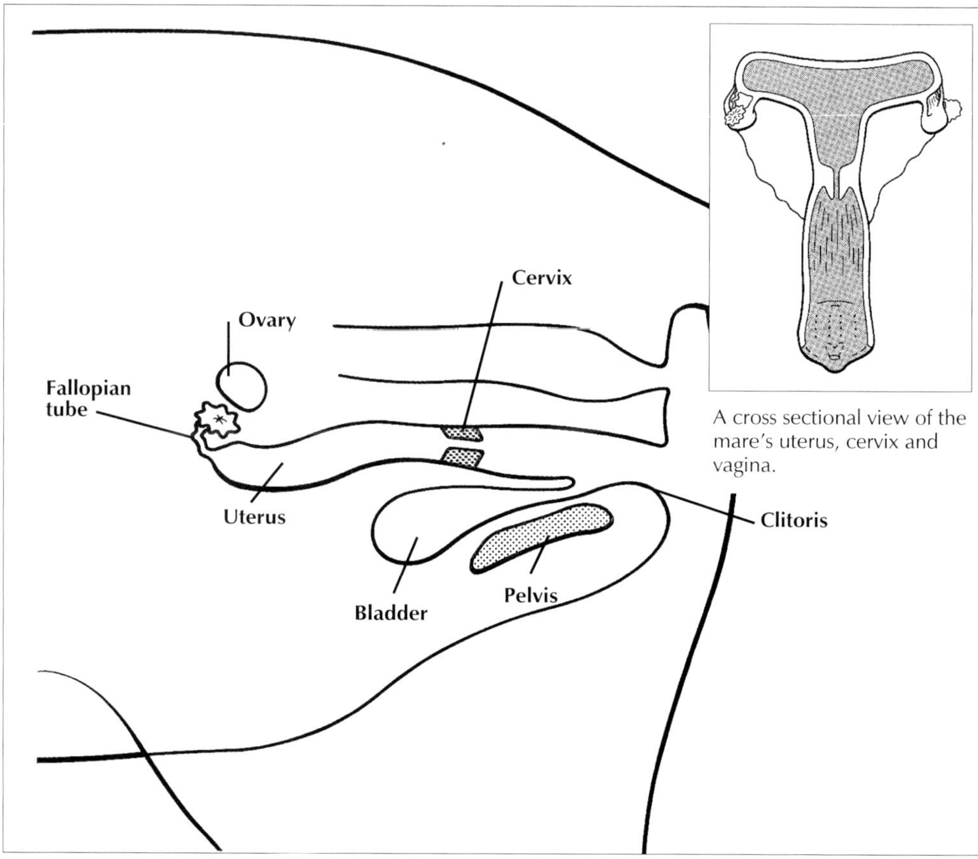

Fig. 95 *The mare's reproductive system*

The female reproductive system

The exterior opening of the mare's reproductive tract is the vulva *(Fig. 95)*. The vulval lips act like swing doors to the rest of the tract, opening when pushed from outside by the stallion's penis during mating and opening when pushed from the inside by a foal at the time of birth. It is important that the vulval lips make a reasonably airlight seal in order to prevent bacteria gaining entry to the rest of the tract, in air or water sucked in from outside.

Inside the vulva is a sort of vestibule called the vagina. In young unmated mares the vagina may have a thin fold of membrane, the hymen, running across from one side to the other and partly blocking the opening of the vagina. On the floor of the vagina is the opening of the urethra, so the vagina marks the meeting of the urinary and the reproductive systems. This opening is next to a small structure called the clitoris, on either side of which is a pocket called a clitoral fossa. The most significant feature of this is that some bacteria can live for many years in these clitoral fossae, even when they have been eliminated from the rest of the body. When we need to test for the presence of such bacteria, we often insert a swab into

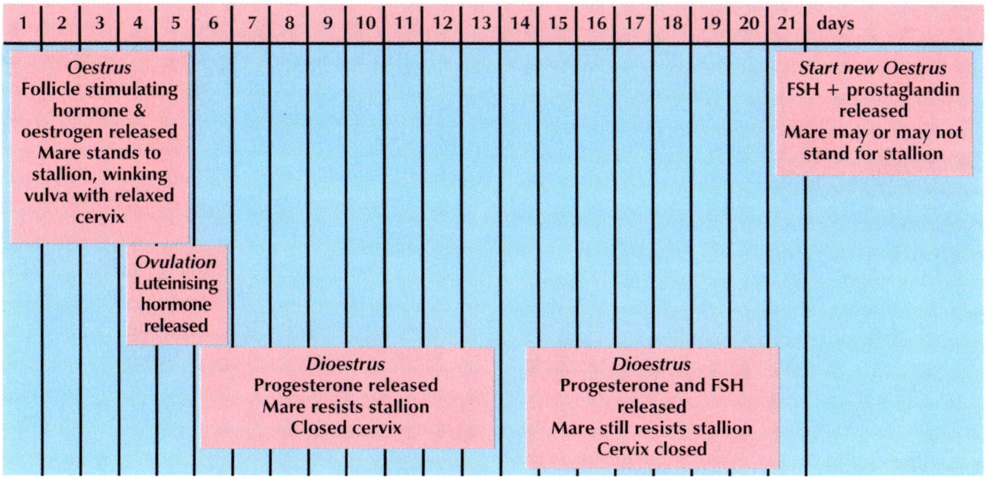

Fig. 96 Hormonal and behavioural changes during the mare's reproductive cycle.

the clitoral fossa. The walls of the vagina have a thin covering of mucus, which contains chemicals to kill off bacteria and so acts as a chemical barrier to disease.

The cervix presents another physical barrier against the passage of infection, further up the reproductive tract. It forms a firm narrow neck in the birth canal for most of the time. But during the mare's season it is softer and more relaxed, and during foaling it is pulled wide open in order to let the foal pass through. When the cervix is wide open after foaling infections can all too easily penetrate deep into the mare.

Beyond the cervix is the uterus, a Y-shaped organ where the foal is carried during pregnancy. The walls of the uterus are relatively muscular, because they are stretched to many times their resting size during pregnancy but must still be capable of contracting forcibly at the time of birth.

Each arm of the Y-shaped uterus ends in a very fine tube called the fallopian tube. Fertilisation of the mare's egg by the stallion's sperm takes place within the fallopian tube. By this stage most of the sperm inserted during mating will have fallen by the wayside. Only the strongest and best sperm will reach the fallopian tube, and usually only one of these will fertilise the egg.

The eggs are released into the fallopian tubes from the ovaries. A mare's ovaries are bean-shaped and approximately 6.5cm (2.5in) long. When a filly foal is born, she already has many thousands of eggs present within her ovaries. When she becomes sexually mature at around two years old, a cycle of activity starts within the ovaries and the body as a whole. A number of eggs, or ova, each become surrounded by a fluid filled sac called a follicle. These follicles increase in size during the mare's period of oestrus, or period of sexual receptivity. Eventually one of the follicles becomes much bigger than the others and moves to a groove on the surface of the ovary which is called the ovulation fossa. The follicle ruptures at the surface of the ovary, releasing the egg to pass into the fallopian tube. This moment is called ovulation. Afterwards the ruptured follicle becomes filled with blood clot and becomes a firm body called a corpus luteum.

Side by side with this ovarian activity we have behavioural changes caused by hormonal activity. As this occurs on a regular cycle, it is called the oestrus or reproductive cycle *(Fig. 96)*. When the follicle increases in size, it does so as a result of high levels of follicle stimulating hormone (FSH). The follicle in turn forms the female hormone, oestrogen. This makes the mare willing to mate with a stallion, to stand for him rather than resisting. Release of a hormone called luteinising hormone causes the follicle to rupture. Ovulation brings oestrus to a close; there is no point in mating if there is no longer an egg available to be fertilized. The corpus luteum formed afterwards secretes progesterone, a hormone which quietens down all activity within the reproductive tract, as well as making the mare unwilling to be mated. Mucus secretion along the tract is reduced and the cervix becomes tight. This is the period of dioestrus, and it lasts approximately 16 days before another follicle starts to enlarge and the whole cycle starts all over again. Mares continue cycling throughout their life, although fertility declines from around 15 years of age.

The cycle does not continue all the year round. In order that the birth coincides with the availability of food and warmth, the mare does not have oestrus cycles during the winter months. During that time there is no activity in the ovaries, and the tract is inactive. The mare is then said to be in anoestrus. The natural breeding season for mares in the northern hemisphere is April to July or August. The thoroughbred industry uses a totally artificial season of 15 February to 15 July, and so fertility is not so good during the early part of that season. In the southern hemisphere the natural mating season is October to January. Some mares still continue to cycle during the winter months, either continuously or for isolated oestrus periods, but they are the exceptions.

In the spring it can take a short while for the mare's reproductive tract to reach full activity. There may be oestrus periods when ovulation does not occur, and the follicle merely subsides again. There may normal cycles without the external signs of oestrus being detectable. There may be irregular cycles. All these are quite 'normal', and usually settle down in time. A mare in oestrus may neigh to attract a stallion's attention. She will stand with her tail raised to one side, exposing her vulva. She will 'wink' the vulval lips, exposing her clitoris when the muscles relax and contract, often passing small amounts of urine at the same time.

Pregnancy

A successful mating results in one of the millions of male sperm penetrating the outer coat of the egg as it passes down the fallopian tube. The two cells combine, so that the resultant foal will have features from both the stallion and the mare. The resulting single cell starts dividing to form a multi-cell embryo. As the number of cells increases, some begin to adopt the characteristics of different types of tissue—for example, skin, bone or nerve cells.

The developing, or foetal, foal has to stimulate some extremely complicated reactions in the mare if it is to survive. First of all, within days of the egg being fertilised, it has to stop the mare coming into season again. What happens is that the corpus luteum does not shrink and fade at the normal time; it maintains its maximum size and its maximum output of progesterone. This prevents the development of further follicles, and also prevents further oestrus periods. Indeed, progesterone has been called the hormone of pregnancy. It maintains the defence mechanisms against infection entering the reproductive tract, and so prevents infection from affecting the foetus.

Sometimes two eggs are ovulated simultaneously. If they are both fertilised, then twin embryos will be produced. This is far more likely to be the cause of twins in the mare than the single fertilised egg splitting into two to produce 'identical' twins. Because of competition for the blood supply in the mare's uterus, twins are rarely the same size at birth.

Even so, the larger twin is often not as big and strong as a normal foal. For this reason many commercial breeders dislike twins and take active steps to prevent them being born. Early pregnancy testing may show the presence of twins and enable steps to be taken to abort both embryos by the use of a drug called prostaglandin, or the manual displacement of one of the embryos per rectum *(Fig. 97)*.

As mentioned earlier, the foal takes approximately 340 days of development before it is ready to be born. During that time it needs to be fed and supplied with oxygen. This is carried to it via the umbilical cord, a tube attached to the foetus's abdomen. The foetal blood comes out along the umbilical vein on the umbilical cord and passes to the placenta, a bag-like membrane which surrounds the foetus but which is so closely attached to the lining of the mare's uterus that oxygen and food substances can pass across from the mare's circulation to that of the foetus. The placenta is the membrane which will later become known as the afterbirth.

As a mammal, the foal is descended from ancestors who lived under water, and so the foal also lives completely surrounded by fluid at this stage. Immediately around the foetus is amniotic fluid, contained by a thin 'bag' called the amnion. Foals are often born with part of this amnion around them, especially over their head. Between the amnion and the placenta is another fluid,

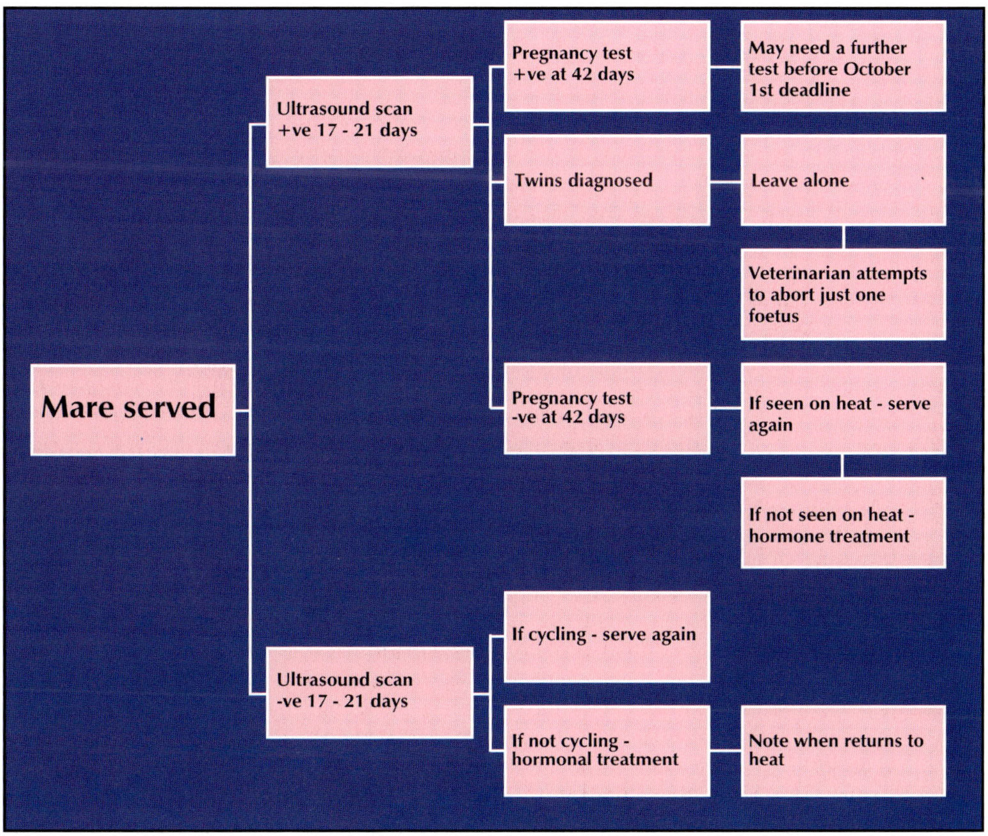

Fig. 97 *Confirming pregnancy in the mare*

the allantoic fluid. This is really the foal's urine which accumulates with time during pregnancy. Although the foal's development may appear to get off to a slow start with the foetus only being around 3cm (1.2in) long at two months after the egg is fertilised, by five months old the foetus looks almost like a 'proper' horse and is 50 - 60cm (20 - 24in) long. At this stage it lies upside down in one horn, or arm, of the uterus.

Breeders are obviously keen to find out whether a mare is pregnant or not. The most superficial way of establishing this is to determine whether the mare has been observed in season since her last mating. If she has, it is unlikely (but not impossible) that she is pregnant. If she has not, then it is possible that she is pregnant, but it might be merely that the observer has not been able to see the signs of heat. The earliest reliable pregnancy detection is at around 17 days after mating, using an ultrasound scanner. This sends out a beam of ultrasound and analyses the resultant echoes. A computer then builds up a picture in which fluid-filled sacs, such as that around the embryo, show as dark areas. From five to six weeks onwards a reliable indication can usually be obtained via an internal examination of the uterus carried out per rectum.

The growing foetus can be felt per rectum as a swelling in the uterine horn which increases in size as the days go by. From 40 days also, a blood sample can be tested for the presence of pregnant mare's serum gonadotrophin (PMSG), a hormone only secreted by the placenta. This last method is not reliable after 110 days of pregnancy, but from that stage onwards the mare's urine can be tested for the presence of another hormone, oestrogen. The mare, more than most other female animals, has a tendency to lose her foetus during the first three months of pregnancy. So a positive early pregnancy test does not always result in a live birth.

Foaling

Although we estimate an average of 340 days for a mare's pregnancy, the length can vary a great deal. Up to one month longer or shorter may still result in a normal term foal. Owners who want to watch the birth of a foal can therefore spend many fruitless nights watching and waiting. Kits are now available which measure the levels of calcium in the mare's milk with a dipstick-type test. These can indicate whether the mare is, or is not, likely to foal during the next 12 hours. If carried out on a regular basis it can reduce the number of sleepless nights for owners. During the week or two before foaling the mare's udder enlarges as the milk-secreting tissue becomes active. This is called 'bagging up'.

One of the first signs that foaling is actually imminent is the appearance of globules of honey-like wax at the tip of the mare's teats. This is called 'waxing up'. and is most noticeable in maiden mares. It may indicate that foaling will occur within the next day or two. Sometimes the mare may produce milk days before foaling, with the result that by the time the foal is born, the vital colostrum, or first milk, which it needs has long since dribbled out of the swollen udder as the mare 'runs milk'. If this happens the foal will not get any immunity against infections. It is therefore worth collecting some of the colostrum and storing it in a deep freeze until the foal is actually born.

We traditionally divide foaling into three stages. During the first stage, the uterus starts to contract. This causes some abdominal pain, so the signs are similar to those of colic. There may be patchy sweating, and the uneasy mare may keep looking round at her flanks. Many mares have false alarms before foaling, especially maiden mares. It may help to recognise these by remembering that most foals are born at night. The first stage of labour normally lasts about two to three hours.

The second stage of labour is the actu-

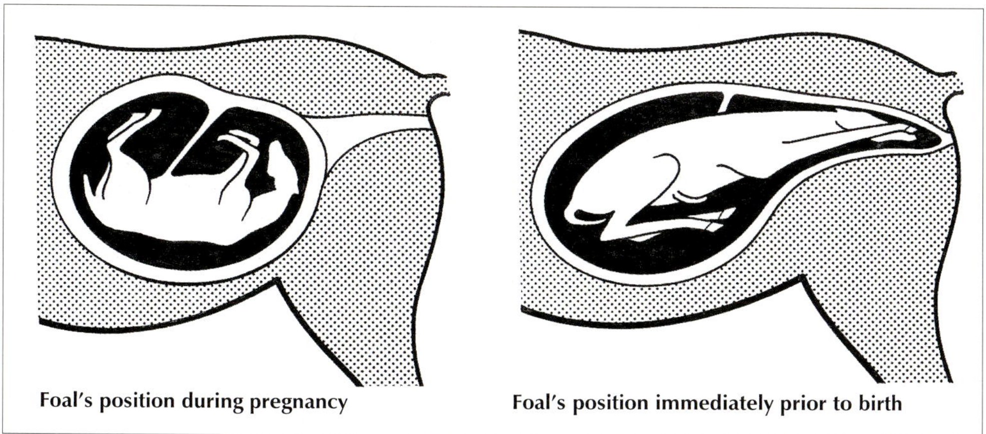

Fig. 98 The position of the foal in the uterus during pregnancy and just before birth.

al delivery of the foal through the birth canal. It usually starts with the bursting of the water bag, or placental membranes, and the release of the allantoic fluid in a rush through the vulva. The mare starts straining forcibly with her abdominal muscles in addition to the unseen uterine contractions. The amnion usually then appears like a pinky-white balloon at the vulva. As the straining becomes more forceful this also ruptures and the foal appears.

Both head-first and tail-first (or breech) births are normal. Whichever it is, both legs need to come through the cervix and pelvic canal alongside each other. When it is an anterior presentation, the head must lie along the forelegs, rather as if the foal was diving out to the outside world *(Fig. 98)*. To have arrived at this position, the foal needs to twist through 180° from the way it lay during most of pregnancy. The contractions in the mare are so very forceful that the birth takes place very quickly, usually within about 20 minutes. Mares rarely have trouble foaling, but when they do, these contractions may aggravate the problem. After the foal has been born, its umbilical cord ruptures. If it does not do so, do not cut or tear the cord because it can continue to pump blood into the foal for some time after birth, and this blood would be lost. If the cord ruptures and haemorrhage occurs, then tie the cord off with a sterile bandage or prepared ligature.

The third stage of labour is the delivery of the placenta. This may be accompanied by some pain for the mare. Normally, the placenta has been pushed out within 10 hours of foaling. It is very important that every last piece of the placenta is expelled, so the placenta should be recovered from the stable or the field and examined fully. It should be Y-shaped, and the two arms of the Y should have sealed, rounded ends *(Fig. 99)*. If the tip of one of the arms appears to have been torn off, every effort should be made to find out whether this happened outside the mare or whether the piece of placenta is still within her.

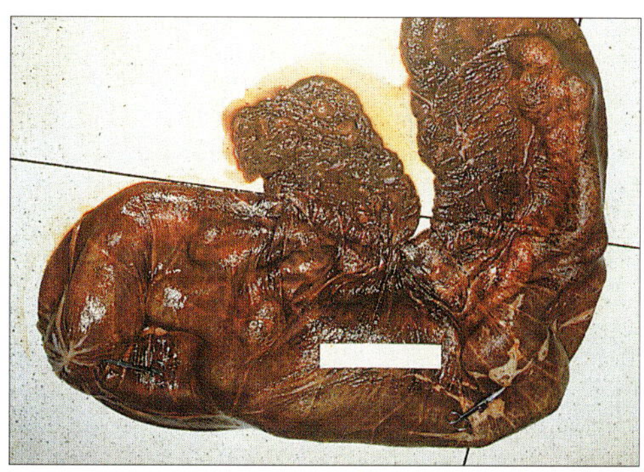

Fig. 99 *The mare's placenta*

The newborn foal

As mentioned earlier, the foal should stand within 20 to 30 minutes. After many false starts it should be suckling within an hour. The mare may need to be restrained to enable the foal to establish suckling. It is vital that the foal gets the adequate colostrum during the first 18 to 24 hours of life, otherwise it will have no resistance to disease at all. It is possible to blood test foals to check that they have absorbed sufficient gamma globulins to provide immunity. If globulins are low a plasma infusion may be necessary, with or without antibiotic cover.

Foaling heat

Most mares come into season around 9 to 10 days after foaling. This heat is called the foaling heat. It is often accompanied by diarrhoea in the foal, which causes concern in novice breeders. The diarrhoea will usually resolve itself without any treatment when the heat period is over. There is often a prolonged dioestrus period between the foaling heat and the next heat period. This has led breeders to concentrate on getting the mare successfully mated during the foaling heat. There are disadvantages, however, in attempting this. At this time the uterus has not fully recovered from the previous pregnancy and foaling. If an infection is introduced into the reproductive tract during the act of mating, then the natural defences may not be strong enough to withstand the infection. This may be one reason why fewer foals are successfully carried to term after foaling heat matings than after later matings. So it is a wise move to wait until the second heat after foaling before mating a mare.

Artificial breeding

Economic pressures sometimes place a strain on traditional breeding methods. A successful competition mare misses the opportunity to add to her winnings for several months if she breeds even one foal. So there is a tendency either to breed from less successful mares, or to delay the start of breeding until the mare is much older, and when her fertility is consequently reduced. For stallions there are limits to the number of fertile matings any one stallion can participate in during the peak natural breeding period. There are artificial solutions for both of these problems, although the resulting foals may not be accepted by the stud book authorities.

A stallion can father more foals by using artificial insemination. This may involve collecting the semen into an artificial vagina during an otherwise normal mating. Some stallions can be trained to ejaculate semen while mounting an 'artifical mare'. Each ejaculation of semen contains enough sperm to ensure a normal fertile mating in several mares. The semen can be divided into portions, to each of which are generally added fluids called extenders to help cushion the sperm against shock and infection. Each semen portion can then be immediately introduced, or inseminated, into the uterus of a receptive mare via a catheter. It is very important that the mare's whole reproductive tract is at exactly the right stage for the sperm to meet and fertilise an egg. This may require considerable veterinary involvement to indicate when to inseminate if there is no stallion to test the mare's reaction.

Stallion semen can also be deep frozen and stored in liquid nitrogen. When such semen is thawed out, the sperm may appear on microscopic examination to be inactive, but they can still be fertile. Artificial insemination (AI) can play a large role in controlling venereal infections that are spread during the act of mating. It also enables semen to be trans-

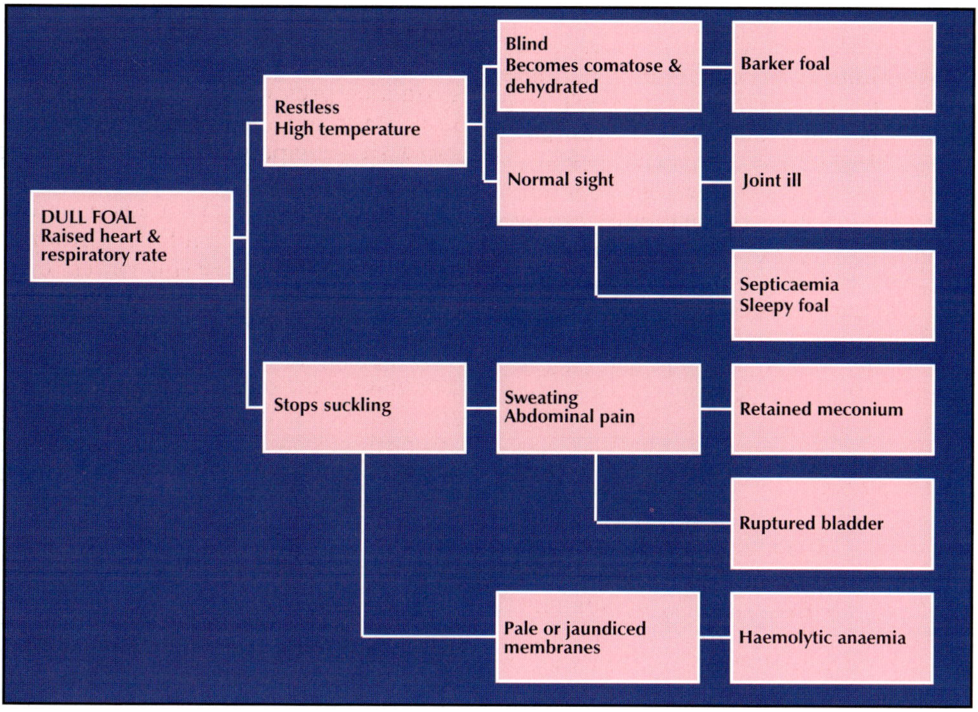

Fig. 100 *The diseases of young foals*

ported from place to place rather than transporting the horses over long distances. AI facilitates breeding from mares that are unable to stand the physical thrusting of natural mating.

Embryo transfer is now becoming commercially available in the horse world. This involves mating a mare and removing the fertilised egg either surgically or non-surgically shortly afterwards. The egg is immediately put into the uterus of another mare, who will carry it to term. This recipient mare has to have had her whole reproductive cycle synchronised with that of the donor mare, so that the egg goes into a fully prepared uterus. Of course, the recipient mare does not need to be of the same quality (or even the same breed) as the donor mare. She simply nurtures and eventually gives birth to the foal while the 'mother' continues performing. Embryo transfer also allows breeding from mares that might, for example, be physically incapable of giving birth to a foal because of injury or other causes.

Disease prevention

Few of the diseases of reproduction can be prevented by specific measures. The horse's general health is, however, of paramount importance because maximum fertility will only be achieved when management, nutrition and freedom from other diseases have all been taken care of. Signs of disease in the young foal are shown above *(Fig. 100)*.

Prevention of infection at the time of mating requires a knowledge of the infective status of both horses. Mare owners must take steps to establish that the stallion has been swabbed and found free from venereal diseases such as contagious equine metritis (CEM) and *Klebsiella* (see pages 97 and 99). They should also seek assurances that no contagious diseases such as EHV1 (see page 51) are present on the stud premises. Stallion owners should receive prior notification that the mare has had a negative clitoral swab for

CEM. In some circumstances they may also require a negative cervical swab, taken when the mare is in oestrus. In view of the fact that EHV1 is basically a respiratory disease which can also sometimes cause abortion, stallion owners should seek an assurance that there is no active respiratory disease at the mare's home stable. Where abortion due to EVA is considered a risk, both stallion and mares should be vaccinated against the disease.

Hygiene is also important at the time of foaling. A clean bed should be available for the mare, and this should be disposed of 24 hours after foaling in order to remove all the discharges which are released at that time. If it is necessary to foal a mare in a box where another mare has recently foaled, it should be thoroughly disinfected between the two foalings.

Abortion

Symptoms Abortion is the loss of a dead foal before the 300th day of pregnancy. If the foetus was quite small, this may not be associated with any other signs from the mare *(Fig. 101)*. If abortion occurs later in pregnancy, the mare may go through the stages of labour associated with normal birth. Abortion is often followed by a vaginal discharge in the mare.

Cause Non-infectious causes of abortion include stress; the failure of the placenta to provide enough nutrition and oxygen for foal growth; twinning, which places too great a demand on the placenta; physical abnormalities of the unborn foal. Infectious causes of abortion may be fungal (e.g. aspergillosis), viral (e.g. EHV and equine viral arteritis), or bacterial (e.g. *streptococcus zooepidemicus*, salmonella or leptospirosis). Low progesterone levels have now been ruled out as a possible cause of abortion.

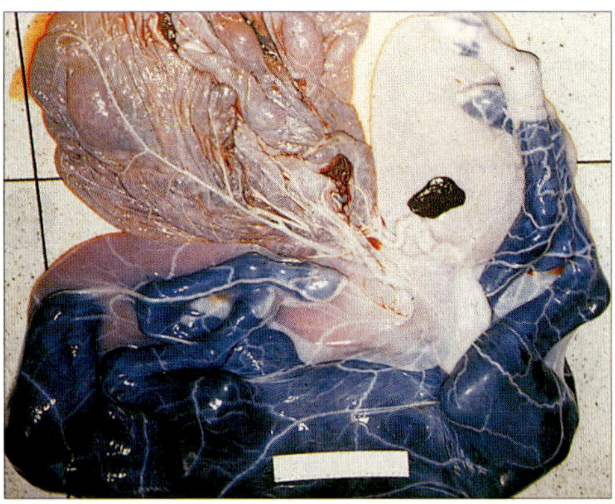

Fig. 101 *An aborted foetus*

Treatment Although treatment of any infection involved may be possible, nothing will save the dead foal. Any infectious cause of abortion must be treated and eliminated if there are not going to be future abortions in the same or other mares.

Prognosis Good.

Anoestrus

Symptoms A mare does not come into season, or oestrus. This is not merely a failure of the visible signs of oestrus—the ovaries are dormant and inactive.

Cause As most mares go into anoestrus during the winter months it is only a pathological problem if it occurs during the breeding season. Anoestrus may follow foaling, or it may be that the cycle simply fails to start in the spring.

Treatment The cycle can be made to occur earlier in the spring by artificially extending the period of daylight. This can be done by using a 200 watt bulb, which should be left on for two and a half hours after sunset, or switched on to provide a one hour light period 9 to 10 hours after sunset. Adding allyl trenbolone to the food daily for 10 days may also cause a rebound into oestrus three to four days after treatment is stopped.

Prognosis Anoestrus cannot usually be overcome in the very middle of winter.

Coital exanthema

Symptoms Can affect both mares and stallions. In both cases small blisters form, which then burst leaving an ulcer *(Fig. 102)*. In the mare the blisters are in the vulva, near the junction between the skin and the pink mucous membrane. In the stallion they are on the penis. When the blisters are forming the horse may be dull and have a fever, but once they burst the horse usually returns to normal. Recovery is usually complete within two to three weeks. Healed ulcers may permanently lose their natural skin pigmentation.

Cause The infection, which is spread during sexual intercourse, is caused by the equine herpes type 3 virus.

Treatment No treatment is necessary for the viral infection, but soothing creams may ease the raw ulcers. Stallions should not be mated for two to three weeks after resolution of the symptoms.

Prognosis Horses cure themselves by the development of natural immunity without any significant effect on their fertility.

Contagious equine metritis (CEM)

Symptoms A venereal disease. Mares may have a profuse vaginal discharge. They return to service much earlier than normal and at irregular intervals. No symptoms may be obvious in the stallion.

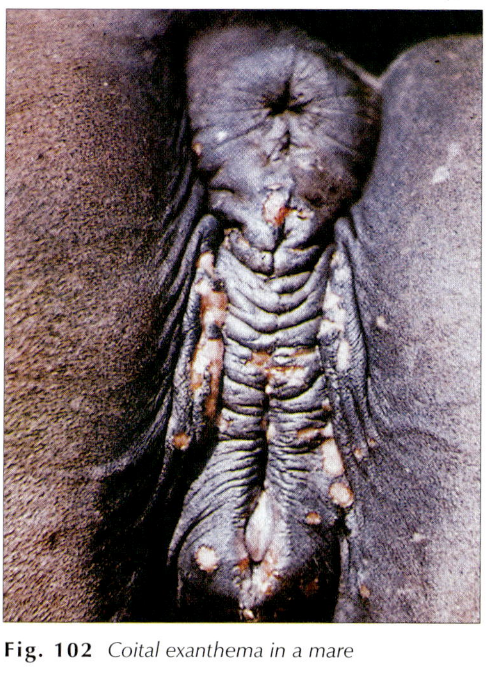

Fig. 102 *Coital exanthema in a mare*

Cause The organism responsible is called *Tayloriella equigenitalis.*

Treatment Local treatment with antibiotics may bring about an apparent cure. There is a strict code of practice to control the disease in thoroughbreds.

Prognosis Both mares and stallions may become symptomless carriers, which can only be detected by anaerobic culture taken from the stallion's penis or the mare's clitoris.

Cryptorchid or rig

Symptoms Cryptorchidism—having a hidden testicle—is probably the commonest physical abnormality of the stallion's reproductive tract. It is a congenital problem. The missing testicle may be held in the inguinal canal which leads into the abdomen, or in the abdomen itself. It can be fertile, and cryptorchids behave like stallions. Owners sometimes suspect that horses which are thought to be geldings but show sexual interest in mares are actually rigs with only the descended testicle removed. A blood test can show whether there is active testicular tissue present if no testicles can be detected.

Cause The condition is due to a failure of development in the foal, as a result of which the testicle does not move out of the abdomen and down into the scrotum. The condition may be hereditary.

Treatment Surgical removal of both testicles should be carried out. This may require a major abdominal operation. It is wrong to only remove the normal testicle; this will not affect what happens to the hidden testicle but may give the false impression that the horse has been castrated. If there is doubt about a hidden testicle, blood hormone levels will indicate the true position.

Prognosis Good.

Dystocia

Symptoms The average time taken for the second stage of labour, when the mare can be seen to be straining to deliver the foal, is about six minutes. If it takes significantly longer dystocia (or difficulty in giving birth) should be considered.

Cause Dystocia may be due to the foal being presented in an abnormal position that prevents it from passing through the birth canal. If only one leg is presented to the cervix and the other one is folded back, or if both legs are presented to the cervix but the head is folded backwards, the foal cannot be born. Dystocia may also be due to the foal having some physical abnormality—it may simply be too big. Dystocia may, on the other hand, be due to the mare's either not straining forcibly enough or failing to open the birth canal sufficiently for the foal to pass through.

Treatment Time is short, so professional help should be summoned immediately. With ample lubrication the foal should be positioned either with both front feet followed by the head, or with both hind legs extended. Reasonable force should then be used to pull the foal out. If it is still not possible to deliver the foal a caesarian section operation may be necessary.

Prognosis Because the mare's uterus usually contracts very forcibly (hence the short time taken by the second stage of labour), a faultily positioned foal may easily cause physical damage to the mare during delivery (see foaling injuries).

False pregnancy

Symptoms The mare fails to come back into oestrus after mating, and gives a positive pregnancy test. If this occurs early in the breeding season, the mare may start cycling again three to five months later, but if it occurs later in the season the mare may not be seen in oestrus again that year.

Cause The mare has indeed been pregnant, but there has been early embryonic death. The 'pregnancy' is maintained either by a persisting corpus luteum, or, after 36 days, by hormones secreted from the placenta.

Treatment The most appropriate method of returning the mare to normal cycling activity will depend on the stage at which the embryonic death occurred. Prostaglandin treatment may remove a corpus luteum, but may be unsuccessful at overcoming the effect of hormone secreted by areas of placental tissue called endrometrial cups.

Prognosis Although cycling activity may not return in time for the mare to be bred from again that breeding season, fertility in future years should be normal.

False rig

Symptoms The horse behaves in many ways like a stallion, attempting to mount mares. No testicles are evident. Blood samples show that no testosterone is actually being produced.

Cause This is a behavioural problem rather than one due to faulty castration.

Treatment No treatment is possible other than discipline.

Prognosis Many of these horses will remain like this all their lives.

Foaling injuries

Symptoms Tearing of the membranes lining the vagina may result in haemorrhage from the vulva which continues long after foaling. Tearing of the vulva and surrounding area is also a relatively common complication after foaling. The result may be an abnormally shaped vulva which allows windsucking.

Cause Such injuries are usually the result of forceful contractions of the uterus overcoming a degree of dystocia and forcing the foal out.

Treatment The repair of the skin tears is usually carried out as part of a Caslick's operation, which temporarily sutures across the upper part of the vulval lips. In all but the most severe cases it is carried out immediately after foaling. In severe, deep wounds however, surgical repair is delayed until the initial inflammation has subsided.

Prognosis As long as the normal anatomy is regained, the mare should be able to foal again. If the tearing is not repaired the mare may become infertile due to the continual establishment of a low grade infection in the vagina.

Granulosa cell tumour

Symptoms The mare may show nymphomania, but may conversely not show any oestrus periods at all. Physically, the mare may develop a marked neck crest and muscles like a stallion. On rectal examination one of the ovaries is markedly increased in size, while the other ovary is small and inactive.

Cause A tumour of granulosa cells in the ovary.

Treatment Surgical removal is the only treatment.

Prognosis After removal, normal activity returns to the other ovary, which is then fertile.

Klebsiella

Symptoms This is a venereal disease. Mares may have a vaginal discharge and return to service at irregular intervals.

Cause There are many strains of *Klebsiella pneumoniae* bacteria, identified by a 'code' of proteins which are present in the capsule around the bacterium. Not all capsular types cause symptoms of disease, so when the organism is isolated from a culture of the vaginal discharge, it is also necessary to find out which type of *Klebsiella* is involved.

Treatment Treatment is difficult. It is essential to use an antibiotic that is active against the specific capsular type of *Klebsiella* present. Treatment should be given to the whole animal, as well as locally into the reproductive tract. Animals should not be bred from again until repeated cultures are negative.

Prognosis The disease may reappear later despite apparent recovery.

Lactation anoestrus

Symptoms The mare fails to come into season again after the foaling heat.

Cause Pregnancy is obviously a possible cause. However, the hormones which support milk production may inhibit the reproductive cycle for some time during early lactation.

Treatment It is obviously necessary to check whether the mare actually is pregnant. No treatment is recommended for true lactation anoestrus because such treatment may interfere with milk production. The possibility of lactation anoestrus is one of the reasons for mating mares at the foaling heat.

Prognosis Mares return to normal cycling activity with time.

Lactation failure

Symptoms The mare stops manufacturing milk while still having a young foal running at foot.

Cause There are many possible causes of lactation failure, including very poor nutrition, systemic illness in the mare and failure of the hormonal system which maintains lactation.

Treatment Once lactation has ceased for a particular lactation, it is unlikely to start again. In any case, by the time artificial means have been found to stimulate milk production the foal may have ceased to rely on its mother's milk.

Prognosis Lactation will probably be normal in future pregnancies.

Mastitis

Symptoms One or both sides of the udder become hard, hot and painful. Pus rather than milk is present in the udder. The mare may have a fever. She may be unwilling to move, and unwilling to allow the foal to suck. Mastitis usually occurs shortly after foaling.

Cause Some element of injury to the teat allows the entry of bacteria into an udder whose resistance to infection is already low. A variety of bacterial species may be involved.

Treatment. Local infusion of an antibiotic into the udder will kill the infection. The abnormal infected secretion should be removed from the udder by hand milking. Systemic treatment of the body as a whole may be necessary. The foal may require bottle feeding to compensate for the loss of milk.

Prognosis Good as long as it is spotted early. Permanent changes in the udder and toxic laminitis (see page 76) may occur if treatment is not carried out successfully.

Nymphomania

Symptoms The mare appears to be permanently in season. All the signs of oestrus are present; indeed, they are often particularly marked even without the presence of a stallion.

Cause Sometimes owners attribute any kind of undesirable behaviour to nymphomania, when there is not any real sexual involvement. Ovarian tumours can cause true nymphomania. 'Cystic ovaries' are also sometimes blamed for the condition, but are not thought to occur in the mare.

Treatment The administration of allyl trembolone in the food for 10 days will dampen down all normal follicular activity and should allow normal heat periods to follow. If an ovarian tumour is present, surgical removal is the only treatment.

Prognosis Good.

Orchitis

Symptoms The testicles are swollen, hot and painful. The stallion may have a raised temperature. It is unwilling to mate.

Cause The inflammation may be caused by trauma, or it may be associated with an infection such as *Streptococcus equi* (the bacteria responsible for strangles—see page 52).

Treatment Cold compresses for the scrotum will help if the stallion will tolerate them. Where infection is involved, systemic antibiotics are needed for a prolonged period until all the swelling has subsided. Rest from sexual activity also needs to be prolonged, and a test mating may be advisable to ensure that full fertility has returned.

Prognosis Guarded for sexual activity.

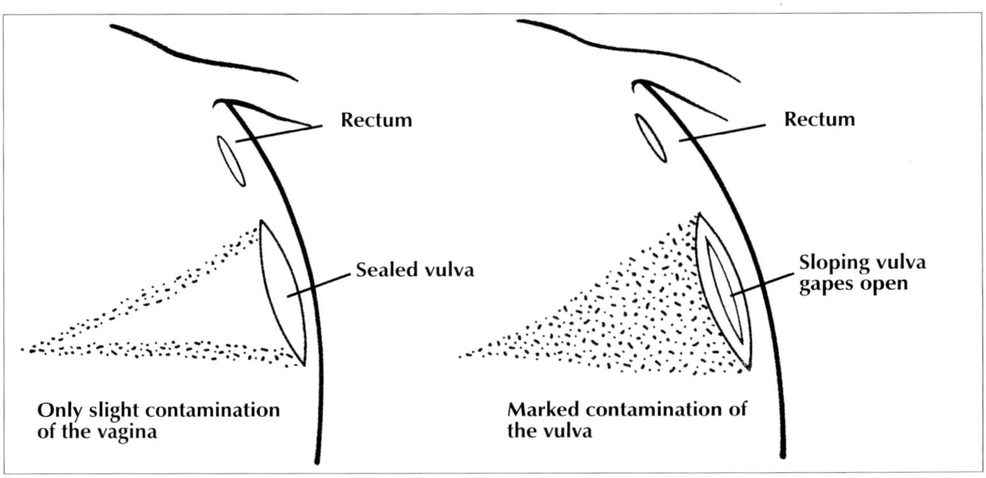

Fig. 103 *Vaginal windsucking in the mare*

Pneumovagina or windsucking

Symptoms Because of faulty anatomy, the lips of the vulva gape open at the top. This allows air (and so infection) to be sucked into the vagina *(Fig. 103)*. The resulting bacterial infection results in the rapid death of any sperm after mating, and the mare keeps returning to service. She may have a slight vaginal discharge.

Cause Relaxation of ligaments with advancing age may allow the vulval lips to fall open. This is especially likely if the mare's conformation results in the lips being anatomically at an angle of 50° or less to the horizontal. Another cause is damage at the time of foaling.

Treatment Caslick's operation sutures the opposing lips of the vulva together, starting at the top of the vulva. If at all possible, sufficient space must be left for the stallion to safely mate the mare. Otherwise the lips must be separated immediately prior to mating and resutured immediately afterwards. The lips must also be separated before foaling.

Prognosis Once a mare develops pneumovagina, a Caslick's operation will usually be necessary after every foaling.

Prolapsed penis (priapism)

Symptoms The penis hangs loosely down from the prepuce and cannot be retracted *(Fig. 104)*. It may become swollen and physically damaged. Where replacement is possible by hand, prolapse recurs when the penis is released.

Cause The condition may be triggered off by overdosage of certain sedative drugs. Trauma may also cause prolapse.

Treatment The penis must be supported in as near a normal position as possible using dressings. Cold water hosing may be beneficial.

Prognosis Guarded.

Prolapsed uterus

Symptoms Shortly after foaling a large, fleshy pink mass is pushed out of the vagina, still attached to the mare.

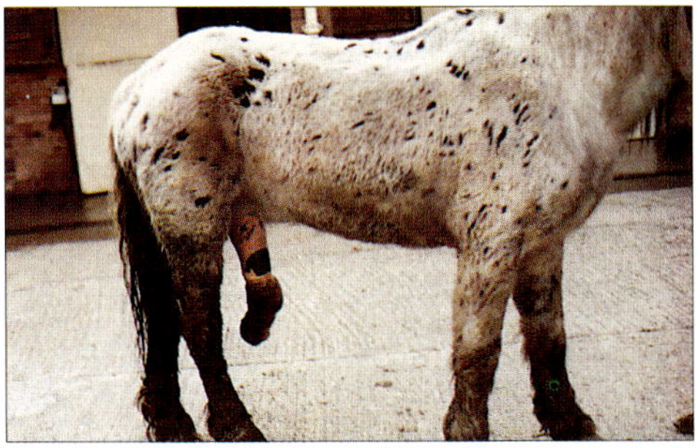

Fig. 104 *A prolapsed penis*

Cause Relaxation of the uterine ligaments and decreased muscle tone due to calcium deficiency are possible causes of the uterus everting through the vagina. The inner lining of the uterus is therefore now the outer covering of the uterine mass.

Treatment The uterus should be kept as clean as possible to prevent infection. Replacement may need epidural, or even general, anaesthesia. The lips of the vulva are sutured to discourage further prolapse. Antibiotic cover controls infection picked up whilst the uterus is outside the body.

Prognosis Shock may follow prolapse of the uterus.

Prolonged dioestrus

Symptoms The mare fails to come into oestrus because she is stuck between oestrus cycles. Rectal examination reveals a corpus luteum in the ovary which fails to decline and allow a follicle to mature ready for oestrus and ovulation. Pregnancy also has a persistent corpus luteum, and must be distinguished from prolonged dioestrus.

Cause The cause is a hormonal imbalance causing high progesterone levels. It is most common in the early spring, between the first couple of oestrus cycles of the year.

Treatment An injection of prostaglandins to effect regression of the corpus luteum and a return to oestrus.

Prognosis Good.

Pseudomonas

Symptoms Those typically associated with an acute infectious endometritis, or inflammation of the uterine lining, including vaginal discharge and early return to service.

Cause The bacterium *Pseudomonas aeruginosa.*

Treatment Local treatment with antibiotics may need to be combined with washing out with silver nitrate solution.

Prognosis It may not be possible to eliminate the condition, and it may be necessary to accept a continuing low level of infection.

Retained placenta

Symptoms The foetal membranes which constitute the placenta are not expelled from the mare's uterus as they normally would be during the first few hours after parturition. The mare develops an increased temperature. Toxic laminitis may follow retention of the placenta.

Cause The membranes fail to separate from the areas of the internal surface of the uterus where they have been exchanging oxygen and food materials during pregnancy. It is usually the non-pregnant horn of the uterus which fails to separate. Twins and premature foalings (including abortions) are likely to be followed by retention of the placenta.

Treatment Physical removal of the membranes should only be attempted when all the attachments have already separated. Otherwise oxytocin (usually via a saline drip) is used to cause separation and expulsion of the membranes.

Prognosis In the past it was considered dangerous to allow the placenta to be retained for more than 12 hours because of the risks of septicaemia (see page 124). The ready availability of antibiotics has greatly reduced this risk.

Silent heat

Symptoms The mare shows no visible signs of oestrus even though her follicles are cycling normally and ovulating.

Cause There are reduced levels of the hormones which cause the visible signs of oestrus (oestrogens) circulating in the bloodstream. Silent heats are especially common early in the breeding season.

Treatment The presence of a stallion may well stimulate more natural signs of oestrus. Mares should be kept in good physical condition. Rectal examination, ultrasound scanning and blood hormone analysis may allow the correct time to mate a mare to be determined even if she is not having obvious oestrus cycles.

Prognosis Good.

Stallion infertility

Symptoms The first sign that a stallion is infertile is that the mares he has mated return to oestrus about 16 days after their previous heat period has ended. Unfortunately other mares will have been mated in the interim, and there is no way of telling so soon after mating whether they are pregnant or not. The ability to successfully impregnate a mare is quite separate from the sex drive to mate or the possesion of apparently normal sexual organs. Sperm abnormalities may be present.

Cause Stallions may be congenitally infertile. More commonly they may be infertile when they first start work due to sexual immaturity. An established stallion of proven fertility may become infertile either temporarily or long-term. Among the factors which may cause this are overwork, inflammation of the testicles, old age and venereal infections such as CEM, *Klebsiella* or *pseudomonas* (see pages *97, 99* and *102*).

Treatment Whatever the cause, the first step is to stop mating any more mares until the problem is solved. Examination of a sperm sample and culture of swabs from the penis may indicate the cause so that specific treatment can be given.

Prognosis Given time most young stallions will become fertile. Acquired infertility has a guarded prognosis.

Umbilical hernia

Symptoms An umbilical hernia is a soft swelling underneath the skin of the ventral abdomen, at the point where the umbilical cord was attached at birth. The swelling disappears with pressure as its contents return into the abdomen.It is usually present from birth or appears shortly afterwards. If a portion of bowel trapped in the hernia is unable to escape, the hernia becomes hot, hard and swollen. The foal then becomes seriously ill.

Cause The hernia is a small sac of abdominal contents which protrudes out under the skin through a hole left where the abdominal muscles failed to fuse before birth. The gap in the muscles does not grow, and so becomes smaller relative to the size of the foal as the foal grows.

Treatment In most cases the hernia is only a blemish, and treatment may not be necessary. Surgery usually involves using a nylon mesh to cover the gap in the muscles and prevent the sac herniating out.

Prognosis Small hernias cause no problems. A large hernia is always liable to become strangulated later and require emergency treatment to replace the trapped intestine.

Virus abortion

Symptoms Abortion after 150 days of pregnancy, especially involving more than one mare (a so-called abortion storm) may be virus abortion. It often follows mild respiratory disease in the horses.

Caus Equine herpes virus type 1 is the usual cause. All the discharges, placentae, etc. are infective.

Treatment No treatment is possible, but vaccination may give some protection. Strict hygiene is essential to prevent further spread. No mares should be allowed to leave the stud during the outbreak. Whenever possible, mares who are still pregnant should be kept separated from aborted or foaled mares to restrict the spread of infection.

Prognosis Good.

8: Diseases of the urinary tract

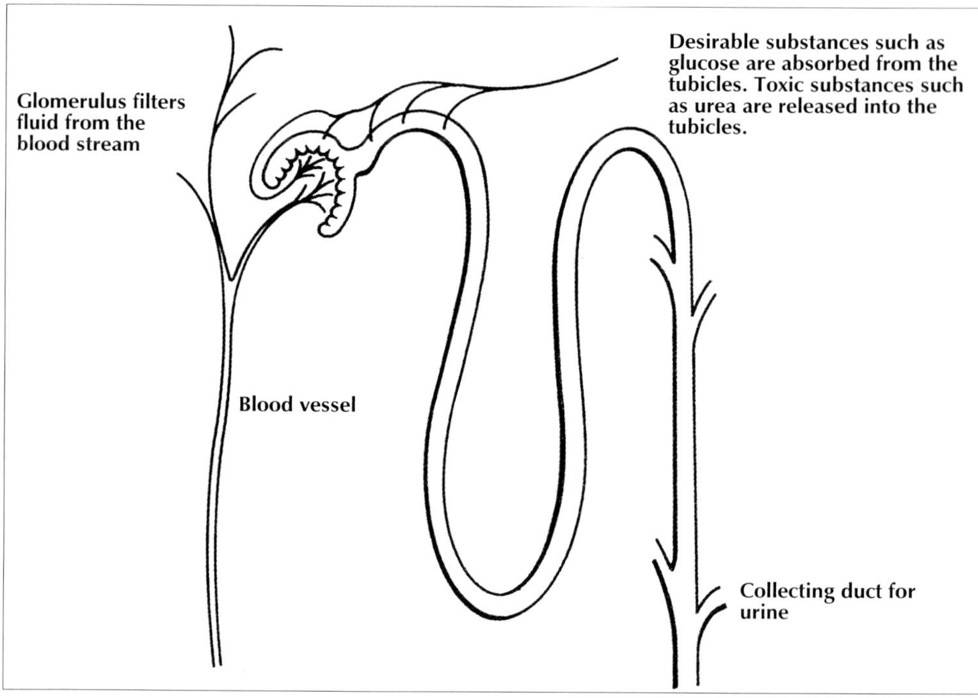

Fig. 105 *The urinary tract*

As blood passes through the kidneys, waste products are filtered from it. About a third of all the heart's output passes through one or other of the kidneys en route to the tissues of the rest of the body, so the blood is at a high pressure as it passes through the clusters of small renal vessels known as the glomeruli. This pressure forces fluid and certain small molecules (but not blood cells or large molecules such as proteins) to pass through pores in the glomerular blood vessel wall and out into a kidney tubule.

Much of the fluid and some other useful constituents which have been filtered out in this way need to be kept because they fulfil a vital role in the body. The filtrate, as the fluid is called, passes along the tubule; the longer the tubule is, the more chance there is for such substances to be absorbed back into the general circulation. The tubules are usually bent back on themselves so that they take up less space and keep the kidney compact in size *(Fig. 105)*. At the end of the kidney tubule, the filtrate (now basically urine) goes into a collecting duct. The kidney is made up of thousands of artery/tubule units. Each one is called a nephron, hence the term 'nephritis' which really just means an inflammation of the nephrons.

It has been estimated that around 500 litres (867 pints) of fluid escapes from the glomeruli of the horse's two kidneys every day. But 495 litres (858 pints) are reabsorbed by the tubules, so that the horse actually produces 5 litres (8.6 pints) of urine per day. Obviously, the control of such large volumes of fluid is crucial to the horse's fluid balance. The rate of water reabsorption is largely controlled by an antidiuretic hormone (which decreases urine output). This is secreted by the pituitary gland, underneath the brain. The level of chemicals in the urine, such as glucose or urea, will depend on the levels circulating in the blood. Abnormal blood levels will stimulate more or less reabsorption in order to restore blood levels to their correct value.

As the continuous flow of urine forms in the kidney, it passes out along a narrow tube called the ureter. This leads to the bladder, where the urine can be stored. An adult horse can store about a gallon of urine in its bladder. The bladder wall is specially constructed in order to allow stretching and contraction as required by the volume of urine it contains. As we look at a horse from the side, the kidneys lie just underneath the vertebral column about two thirds of the way along the back. The bladder lies just in front of the pelvis on the floor of the abdomen.

The passage of urine from the bladder out of the horse depends on the horse's sex. In mares it has only to pass along a short 7.5 to 10cm (3 - 4in) urethra into the vagina. In male horses it has to pass along a quite long urethra which extends out of the abdomen, over the back of the pelvis and forward under the skin to the penis. This has practical considerations because male horses are far more likely to retain their urine in the bladder when they feel abdominal pain from any cause, such as colic, than are females. This is basically because the anatomy of the urethra is more complicated in the male than in the female.

The character of a horse's urine can cause needless concern to owners. Horse urine is usually much more cloudy than human urine because it contains much larger amounts of calcium carbonate crystals. Feedstuffs which are rich in calcium, such as alfalfa, are particularly associated with cloudy urine. If large amounts of body pigments—e.g. haemoglobin from blood or myoglobin from muscles—are being broken down elsewhere in the body, then these pigments will be excreted in the urine and will alter its colour by making it reddish-brown. Because the majority of unwanted substances are eliminated via the urine, analysis of a urine sample is often a major part of any programme for detecting unlawful substances that may have been administered to the horse.

For reasons which will be obvious after considering how urine is formed from the bloodstream, such substances can often be detected in the urine even after they can no longer be found in the blood. Blood levels of electrolytes such as sodium, calcium and magnesium are usually maintained at a fairly constant level, and so measuring them does not provide much information on their levels in the rest of the body. Urine levels may be significant, but obviously vary depending on the concentration of the urine. In conditions such as azoturia where electrolyte levels may be significant a creatinine clearance test is carried out. This compares urine levels with the blood levels using the levels of naturally occuring creatinine (which are remarkably constant) as a reference point.

By and large, urinary problems are relatively rare in the horse compared with other species. Horse owners often have a false impression of the likelihood of kidney problems being involved in weight loss in the horse. They also tend to attach too much importance to changes in the actual physical characteristics of the urine.

Disease prevention

Owners are sometimes under the impression that the higher the protein content of a feed, the better it is. This is not necessarily the case. High protein intake leads to demands on the kidneys which are responsible for excreting the surplus.

Certain chemicals act as diuretics, causing the horse to manufacture an increased amount of urine. If you are not aware of this you may think wrongly that the horse actually has a urinary problem. A high level of salt in the diet, derived from excessive consumption of salt licks, has this effect. The most commonly used diuretic veterinary drug with this effect is frusemide. Certain drugs put an extra strain on the kidneys during their metabolism, so veterinary surgeons may not feel it is safe to use them even though they may be effective against the primary disease. This is especially the case in old horses where age might already have reduced kidney function.

Cystic calculi

Symptoms The horse continually strains to pass urine, but without success. There may be blood in the urine. The horse may appear to have colic.

Cause Calculi, or stones, are formed by the precipitation of mineral salts in the urine. They block the flow of urine out into the urethra.

Treatment Surgical removal is the only long term treatment, but temporary relief is obtained by passing a catheter into the bladder and withdrawing the urine.

Prognosis Guarded. The problem may recur.

Cystitis

Symptoms The horse strains frequently, but only produces small volumes of urine. Urination itself appears to be painful. The frequent dribbling of urine may scald the skin. The problem is more common in mares.

Cause Cystitis is an inflammation of the bladder caused by an infection with a range of bacteria. There may, however, be an underlying cause which has lowered the horse's resistance.

Treatment Systemic antibiotic treatment will kill the bacteria in time but it must be kept up for a long time. Up to four weeks treatment may be needed in chronic cases.

Prognosis When an untreated underlying cause remains, the problem may recur.

Leptospirosis

Symptoms Jaundice is the most obvious symptom, affecting the 'pink' membranes of the mouth, eyes, nose, etc. Care must, however, be taken because the mucous membranes of the horse's mouth are naturally more yellow than those of a human being. The horse has a fever, and is very dull. Pregnant mares may abort. The organism responsible may be cultured from the urine. Antibody levels may be measured in the blood.

Cause Leptospira organisms infect the kidney. They can spread the disease to man.

Treatment Penicillin and broad spectrum antibiotics can kill the leptospires.

Prognosis Good as long as no physical damage is caused to the kidney, for example, fibrosis of the tubules.

Nephritis

Symptoms The general symptoms of nephritis, or inflammation of the kidneys, are increased thirst and urination, but this might not be noticed in horses out at pasture. The horse may go off its food and start to lose weight, and this will be noticed. Blood samples will show a raised blood urea level.

Cause There are a large number of possible causes of nephritis, but it must affect more than one kidney to produce symptoms because there is a large safety margin in the urinary system. Some drugs and other chemicals can cause nephritis following very high doses.

Treatment Fluid therapy can compensate temporarily for the upset fluid balance in the body. Anabolic steroids reverse the weight loss, which is due to using proteins from muscles to replace those lost in the urine.

Prognosis Physical damage to the kidneys often does not heal, and nephritis can become a chronic problem.

Patent urachus

Symptoms This is a condition of foals. The main symptom is that urine drips from the navel. This is most obvious when the foal attempts to urinate, in which case urine comes from both the navel and the urethra (i.e. through the penis in a colt or the vagina in a filly). The skin around the navel can become badly scalded due to the urine. Sometimes infections become established on this inflamed area, and these can then spread internally.

Cause During its foetal life the foal has a tube called the urachus which drains urine from the bladder and takes it to the umbilical cord. This tube normally seals at birth. If it does not do so, it is said to be a patent urachus.

Treatment Sometimes the problem solves itself because the urachus eventually closes. If not, caustic agents may be used (with great care) to cauterise the opening of the urachus. If all else fails, surgery may be needed to tie off the urachus. In all cases the dermatitis due to scalding will need treatment both to kill off infection and to prevent further scalding.

Prognosis Good. Failure to notice the problem may allow a bladder infection (cystitis) to become established which may be troublesome to treat.

Rupture of bladder

Symptoms This is usually a condition seen in young foals, especially colts. The foal becomes dull two to three days after birth, and stops suckling. It may show signs of colic. Its abdomen gradually becomes swollen with fluid. Careful watching reveals failure to pass urine normally. Tapping gently on the side of the foal's abdomen gives the impression that it is like a balloon filled with liquid.

Cause The condition is traumatic in origin, although it may occur as a result of excess abdominal pressure during the birth process. The higher incidence in colts is thought to be due to the fact that the relatively long male urethra cannot empty the bladder quickly enough to compensate for the great pressure on the foal's abdomen as it passes through the mare's pelvis. The rupture usually occurs on the top surface of the bladder.

Treatment Surgery is the only real answer to the problem. Initially, the urine may be drained out of the abdomen while efforts are made to get the foal fit enough to withstand anaesthesia.

Prognosis Until the foal has successfully recovered from the anaesthetic, the prognosis must always be guarded. This is because of the toxic effects of the leaked urine on the other abdominal organs. Once the bladder has been successfully repaired, however, the prognosis is good. The bladder wall heals well.

9: Diseases of the skin

Whenever you walk into a large department store it seems that most of the ground floor is given to female beauty products. Large sums of money are spent on human skin care every year. Yet we do not always pay so much attention to our horse's skin.

When we look at a healthy horse in summer with a gleaming summer coat, there is a great deal our eyes cannot see. The skin, or epidermis, is made up of many layers of cells and lies on top of a fibrous layer called the dermis. Only the cell layers at the bottom of the epidermis are alive and multiplying. The cells in the surface layers are dead. The thickness of the skin is, to a large extent, determined by how many layers there are. Horses have a relatively fine skin, with a few layers of dead cells (which become impregnated with a protective protein called keratin) on the top. The underlying dermis provides support for the epidermis, and contains blood vessels, hair follicles and glands.

When a skin wound is sutured, the aim is to bring the two edges of epidermis together so that they can join to one another. If a wound is left unstitched, it will remain as raw tissue until the epidermis from the surrounding skin has spread across the wound and completely covered it. This is because skin wounds heal in either of two ways. Ideally, they should heal by 'first intention'. This means that there are two clean, uninfected edges which either already lie in contact with each other or can be made to do so by suturing.

In this situation the epidermis literally bridges the gap and seals the break. This is a rapid form of healing, with the wound being sealed by the fourth day after it was formed, and able to withstand normal tension and movement by about ten days afterwards. Ideally, all surgical wounds should heal by first intention healing.

Where the skin edges are separated by a significant gap, or where they are damaged, or where they are infected, the healing has to take place by 'second intention'. This involves the formation of granulation tissue to fill the gap between the skin edges. This granulation tissue contracts over a period of weeks, and eventually the epidermis slowly grows over the top of it to obliterate the wound. Wounds which heal by second intention are far more likely to result in scarring than those which heal by first intention. They also take very much longer to heal.

Horse skin wounds, especially those of the lower limbs, have a great tendency to form proud flesh when they are healing *(Fig. 106)*. This is a property of granulation tissue, which is really a mass of collagen fibres and blood vessels with little ordered structure. Once the granulation tissue increases enough to push through the wound and above the level of the surrounding epidermis, it tends to prevent any more healing. So what starts off as a very sensible attempt to form a tissue which will quickly fill in the deficit caused by the wound becomes a positive hindrance to proper healing. So far attempts to control proud flesh have relied on its physical removal by surgery, freezing, cautery or chemical means (usually based on copper sulphate). There is a suggestion that its formation is mediated by a substance called serotonin, and that there may be a means of persuading the body to remove the granulation tissue by the use of drugs which counteract the serotonin.

The horse's skin comes under assault from a number of different types of living organism, including the spores of fungi (such as ringworm) and bacteria. Of course, there are natural defences. Oily

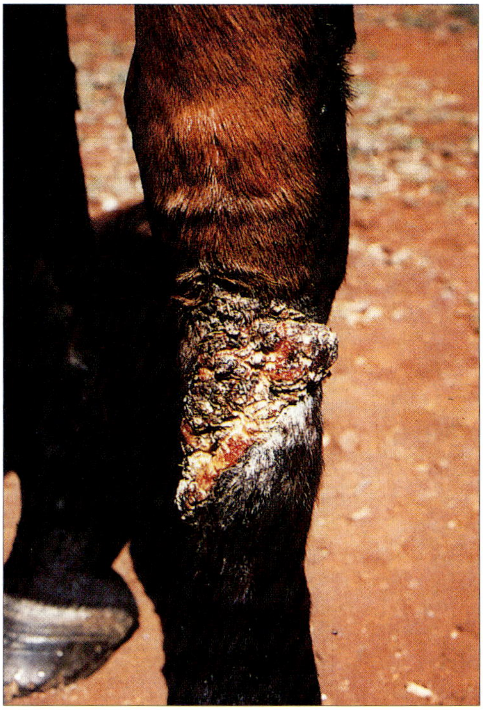

Fig. 106 *Infected granulation tissue*

secretions from the skin glands contain substances toxic to bacteria, and the keratinisation of the surface cells makes them tough and not easily damaged.

Once the horse has become infected, the question has to be asked whether that particular horse now poses a threat to other susceptible horses. There is a distinction between something being contagious and something being infectious. A contagious disease can only spread from one horse to another if the two animals come in direct contact with each other. An infectious disease can spread from one horse to another without there being direct physical contact. So all infectious skin diseases are also contagious, but not all contagious diseases are infectious because if the horses are separated by even a short distance, the infection cannot spread.

In practice, the two terms tend to be treated as if they are interchangeable. For example, ringworm may be said to be contagious because it can be spread by physical contact between two horses, but it can also be spread indirectly via stable walls, fencing or tack; so strictly speaking it is infectious rather than contagious.

It is perhaps worth taking a general look at natural and man-made defences against parasites, fungi and bacteria.

Lice live on the skin all year round, although they cause more irritation during the winter than at any other time, because the thick winter coat provides shelter for them to move around. Secondly, they are more active at low temperatures. Keeping a horse clipped deprives the lice of their shelter, and so reduces their activity. If your horse needs its winter coat, you should dust the horse with louse powder every month or so during the winter. Louse powder is cheap, and prevention is better than seeing the amount of damage a louse-infected horse will inflict on itself. Ivermectin, which is used to control gastrointestinal worms, is also effective at killing lice because it permeates the skin and is therefore taken in by the louse every time it bites the horse.

Keeping ringworm at bay is more difficult. Lice cannot live for any length of time away from the horse, and infestation can be controlled by killing them on the horse's body. Ringworm spores, on the other hand, can survive for more than a year away from the horse. Spores which one horse rubs on to a fence or stable will remain infective for a long time and then be picked up by another horse. Also, it may be three months before the spores on the skin cause visible symptoms.

There are no long-term dressings which will kill ringworm spores on contact, and antibiotic washes, which are effective in the short term, cannot be applied as a prophylactic to prevent future re-infection. The only preventive measures you can take are to avoid contact with infected horses. Unfortunately some irresponsible owners, owing to poor powers of observation, continue to take horses with perhaps one or two ringworm lesions to places where they will meet other, susceptible horses.

However, if a horse has completed a seven-day course of griseofulvin treatment and had a wash with an anti-fungal antibiotic, it is safe even if there are still visible lesions.

Of course, you must not only avoid direct contact with infected horses. Any tack, riding gear or grooming equipment from an affected horse must also be avoided.

All animals co-exist quite happily with the millions of bacteria living on their skin, most of which do not cause disease. Some of them, *Dermatophilus congolensis* being a common example, can cause trouble if they penetrate the top layers of the skin. Mud fever and rain scald, which may both be caused by *Dermatophilus,* are basically controlled by efficient stable management. Although you cannot prevent your horse's lower legs from getting wet, you can prevent them remaining wet. Dry the legs whenever you return to the stable. This helps to prevent the superficial layers of skin becoming waterlogged and vulnerable.

When mud fever first becomes established it forms a small crust. This protects the infection from drying out (and also from most of the ointment which you might apply). The crust largely relies on the skin hairs for stability *(Fig. 107)*. Thick hair at the heels and down the back of the pastern poses more of a threat from providing a cover for mud fever than its removal does from leaving the skin surface less protected. If mud fever establishes even a small area of infection, the whole of the area should be completely clipped out.

Bacterial skin infections are often perpetuated by rubbing from tack or rugs. These same items can carry the infection from day to day, or even horse to horse, so from time to time they should be washed in mild antiseptic.

The skin fulfils a vital function in getting rid of heat produced in the body during exercise. The heat is basically transferred from the deeper tissues (such as the muscles) via the bloodstream. That is why the blood vessels of the skin become so prominent during exercise, allowing the air to cool the blood. Most of the heat, however, is lost via sweat. Sweating can cool the horse even when the environmental temperature is greater than the horse's body temperature. Sweat is formed in sweat glands all over the horse's body, although there are greater concentrations of them in areas such as the neck. The glands themselves are down in the dermis, next to the hair follicles.

Sweat is not just water. It contains large amounts of electrolytes, or salts, and proteins. These proteins act rather like detergents in that they help to disperse the sweat in a thin film along the hairs rather than leaving it in droplets. They are also responsible for the lathering of sweat

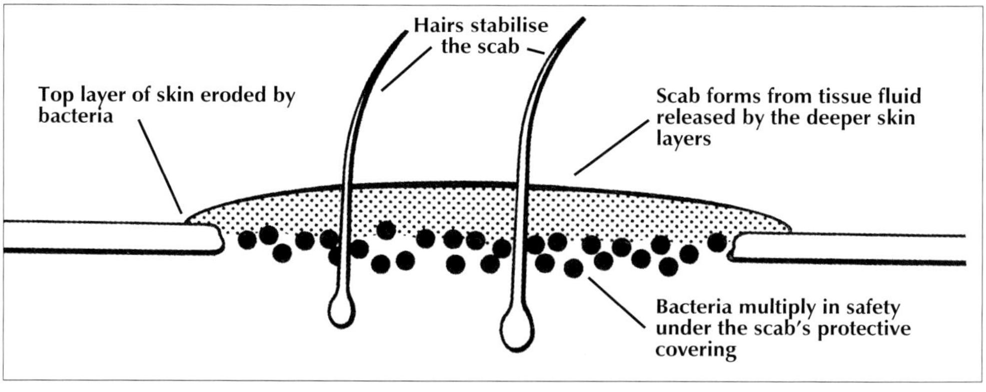

Fig. 107 Diagram showing the effects of mud fever on the horse's skin.

which occurs in horses but not in human beings. The more the horse sweats, the lower the concentration of protein in the sweat and so the more watery the sweat becomes.

The actual cooling is achieved by the evaporation of the sweat. Every litre of water which evaporates removes 580 kilocalories of heat, and a horse carrying out steady work in cool conditions can lose 7.5 litres (13 pints) of sweat per hour. Unfortunately the higher the environmental humidity, less evaporation takes place. The horse will still sweat, but the sweat literally just runs off the horse and has very little cooling effect. This is why in an emergency situation veterinarians may use air blowers on exhausted horses after very strenuous exercise—every drop of sweat which drops off the horse is a wasted opportunity to cool it down. Sweat rugs hold the sweat next to the skin to give it a better chance of evaporating.

Disease prevention

Regular grooming is vital for the prevention of skin disease. When carried out vigorously, it stimulates the circulation to the skin. Grooming removes dirt which might otherwise contaminate tiny scratch wounds, and also removes grease and scurf which can 'clog up' the skin pores. Perhaps most importantly though, grooming forces you to look at the skin over the whole of the body, so ensuring that any problem which does arise may be spotted straight away. Note that grooming equipment can spread disease if it is used on several horses without disinfection between each one.

Many horses are clipped in the winter months. The aim is to increase the rate of heat loss after strenuous exercise by making sweating easier. Sweating onto a thick winter coat, and leaving the sweat to dry there, produces matting of the coat which can seal in and protect infections. Clipping helps to keep such infections at bay, as well as making their detection easier. Unfortunately, even when expertly done, clipping causes minute scratches on the skin surface. When performed by inexperienced hands it can produce obvious grazes. These provide an entrance for infection until healing begins, so a recently clipped horse should never be turned out in the rain, nor dressed with a dirty rug. Regular cleaning and disinfection of the clipper blades during the clipping will help to prevent the spread of any existing infection from one part of the body to another. It is also worth remembering that sharp clipper blades do the job more quickly and with less damage to the skin.

Tack is a common cause of skin problems. Badly-fitting tack rubs the skin and can cause open sores. At the same time one of the commonest reasons for tack not fitting properly is that it belongs to another horse, providing a way of cross-infection. The best way to prevent such problems is for each horse to have its own tack.

The greatest aid to equine skin care is observation. Skin problems rarely explode, they increase gradually. Nip them in the bud *(Fig. 108, see over page)*.

Anhydrosis

Symptoms The horse fails to sweat at all, even in circumstances when it would be expected to do so; or shows markedly reduced sweating. The skin is very dry and scurfy. The symptoms often appear shortly after a move to hotter climates, but the condition can occur in temperate climates. As might be expected the horse is lethargic and takes a long time to recover after exercise.

Cause In most cases the condition is caused by the exhaustion of the sweat glands, which reach the stage where they cannot produce any sweat at all.

Treatment There is no specific medication. The horse should be kept in a cool

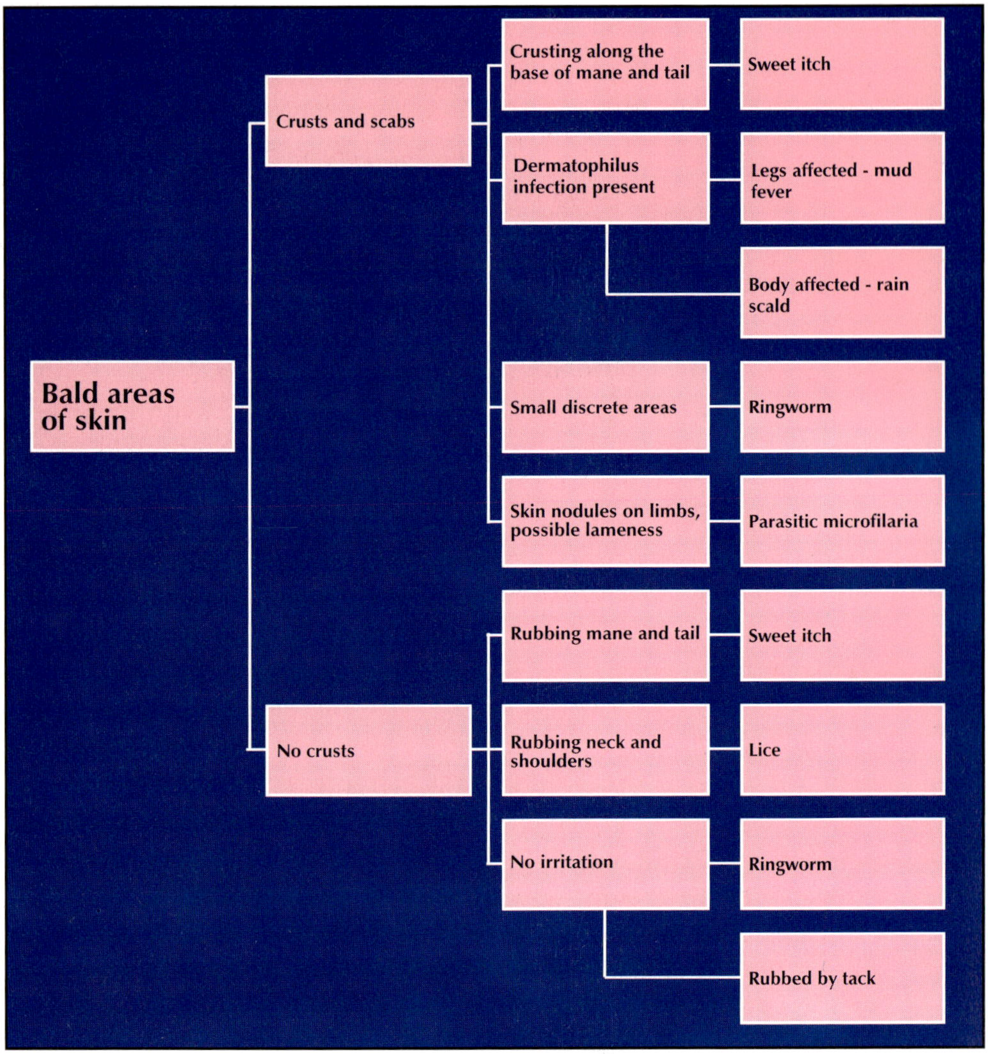

Fig. 108 *Causes of hair loss in the horse*

or air-conditioned climate if possible and exercise avoided in the hope that some of the sweat glands will recover. Shampooing, especially with benzoyl peroxide, may ease some of the discomfort caused by the build up of scurf.

Prognosis Once affected, horses seldom recover.

Burns

Symptoms An intensely inflamed area of skin may be covered by either fluid-filled blisters or a sheet of dead skin. If the blisters burst, or the sheet of dead skin is removed, the raw tissue underneath may become secondarily infected.

Cause Dry heat such as a flame.

Treatment Whenever possible air should be excluded from burns. This is done both to prevent loss of body fluids through the raw tissue and to prevent infection. At the moment of formation burns are, of course, sterile. Non-adherent dressings must be used. Oily ointments should not be applied to burns without veterinary supervision. Cortisone, both topically and by injection, reduces the inflammation. Skin grafts may be required if healing does not take place.

Prognosis Healing of burns is usually accompanied by a degree of scarring. When large areas of the skin are involved the toxic shock and fluid loss involved can be fatal.

Cellulitis

Symptoms There is extensive skin oedema, usually spreading up the affected leg. The skin may be warm to the touch. Close investigation will reveal a break of some kind in the skin surface. The swelling tends to improve with exercise, but recur with resting *(Fig. 109)*.

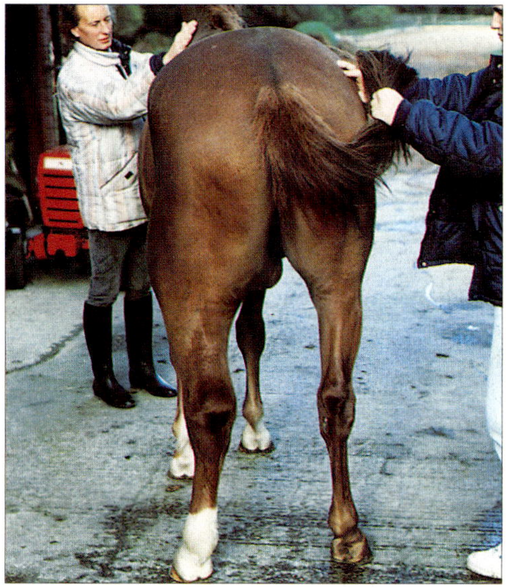

Fig. 109 A swollen leg due to cellulitis.

Cause Cellulitis is an infection of the loose connective tissue between the dermis and the underlying tissues. A variety of infectious organisms can be involved, but there has always been prior injury of some kind to allow the infection to gain entry to these deeper structures.

Treatment Systemic antibiotics will kill the infection, although treatment often needs to be continued for some time. If the blood vessel walls have been damaged, oedema will contine to accumulate when the horse is not active for long periods after the original cause has been overcome. This is because the damaged blood vessel walls allow tissue fluid to escape faster than it can drain away.

Prognosis Prognosis is good once an antibiotic has been found to which the infection is sensitive.

Habronemiasis (summer sores)

Symptoms Raised and ulcerated areas can develop around open wounds, the eyes or the tip of the penis *(Fig. 110)*. The ulcerations do not heal. When they are around a wound, it may look as if the wound has formed some proud flesh, or granulation tissue.

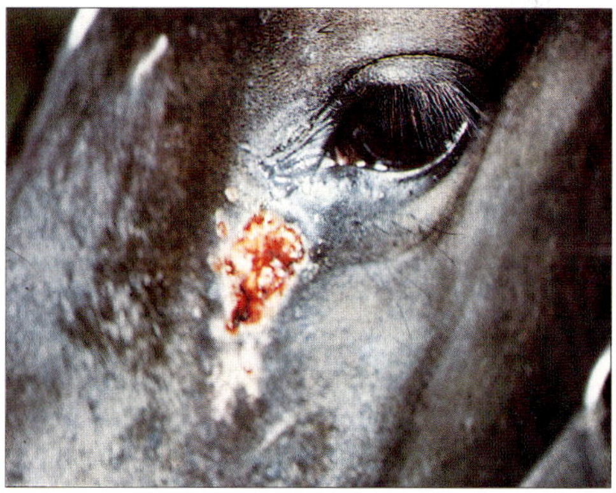

Fig. 110 Habronemiasis around a horse's eye.

Cause Habronema is a stomach worm, although it causes few internal symptoms. The skin ulcerations are due to Habronema larvae. These escape from the mouthparts of flies (such as the stable fly or the house fly) as they land on moist areas of the horse's skin. They stimulate a very acute reaction in the skin before migrating internally.

Treatment Ivermectin is very effective at killing off both adult worms in the stomach and larvae in the skin. Cortisone preparations may then help speed up the resolution of the inflammatory reaction in the skin. If secondary bacterial infection has taken place, topical antibiotic treatment will be needed. Large lesions can be removed surgically.

Haematoma

Symptoms A haematoma is a soft blood-filled swelling under the skin. The swelling usually comes up quite rapidly, and then stays the same for several weeks. The swelling is not painful and is not associated with heat or any apparent illness. It needs to be differentiated from other cases of swelling such as abscesses, by seeing whether clear bloody fluid escapes from a needle inserted into the swelling. A haematoma does not pit on pressure in the way that a localised oedema does.

Cause The vast majority of haematomas are due to trauma of some kind. The trauma ruptures a blood vessel underneath the skin, and bleeding occurs (hence the name, derived from the Greek word for blood, haematos, and -oma, indicating a tumour or growth) until the blood under the skin is under sufficient pressure to stop any more escaping from the blood vessel.

Treatment Just draining the blood out of a haematoma (because it is not in contact with external air it does not clot in the normal way) only allows more haemorrhage to occur. It may be possible at some sites to drain the haematoma and apply firm pressure to the skin so that there is no longer a potential space into which fresh bleeding may occur. Frequently, however, this is unsuccessful. Ultrasound and vibratory massage may speed the disposal of the blood. In some cases the haematoma has to be drained surgically, leaving a sufficiently large hole to prevent clotting trapping any further blood inside the haematoma. In most cases the haematoma is best left at least two weeks before surgical drainage in order to allow some possibility of clotting or sealing of the damaged blood vessel.

Prognosis Left alone the fluid will eventually become organised, or clotted, and the fluid part will be resorbed. Some swelling will remain. This process may take a couple of months.

Harvest mites

Symptoms Irritation of the skin where the mites are living. Hairs are broken off and the horse rubs itself, possibly even causing raw areas of skin.

Cause The harvest mite, *Trombicula autumnalis,* is only an occasional skin parasite of the horse, being picked up from vegetation. It is commonest in the late summer and autumn. The mites are just about visible to the naked eye as moving pink specks, but they are more reliably seen by examining scurf which has been brushed from the skin under a magnifying glass.

Treatment There are a number of anti-parasite washes available which can be used, for example benzene hexachloride or bromocyclen. Treatment needs to be carried out weekly for at least four weeks. If the horse returns to the site where it picked up the original infestation, the problem may return.

Prognosis Good.

Mange mites

Symptoms Small nodules form around the burrows which mites make into the horse's skin. The hair may fall out of the skin over the nodules as a result of the horse rubbing affected areas to relieve the intense irritation it feels. Where the skin surface is rubbed, scabs may be formed. There are three main mites involved, and each tends to affect particular areas of the body. *Psoroptes equi* is common on the poll, mane and tail *(Fig. 111)*. *Chorioptes bovis* is usually found below the knees and hocks *(Fig. 112)*. *Sarcoptes scabei* will affect the neck, shoulders, head, chest, flank and abdomen.

Cause The three mange mites mentioned are microscopic parasites of the skin.

They lay their eggs in the burrows under the skin every day of their short 12 to 15 day adult life. The eggs hatch in four days and the mites take about 10 to 14 days to reach maturity. Diagnosis is confirmed by examining skin scrapings from the affected areas under a microscope.

Treatment Strenuous efforts should be made to dislodge all the scabs with stiff brushes and washing. The whole skin surface should be thoroughly treated with drugs such as coumaphos. Ivermectin given as an oral paste may also be of value. All treatment should be repeated at least twice at seven-day intervals. Because the mites can be transmitted by contact with infected horses, blankets and grooming kit, it is important to separate infected horses. Grooming kit should be cleaned with boiling water, or with the same chemical as is used on the horse.

Prognosis Good. In some countries this is a notifiable disease which should be reported to the relevant authority.

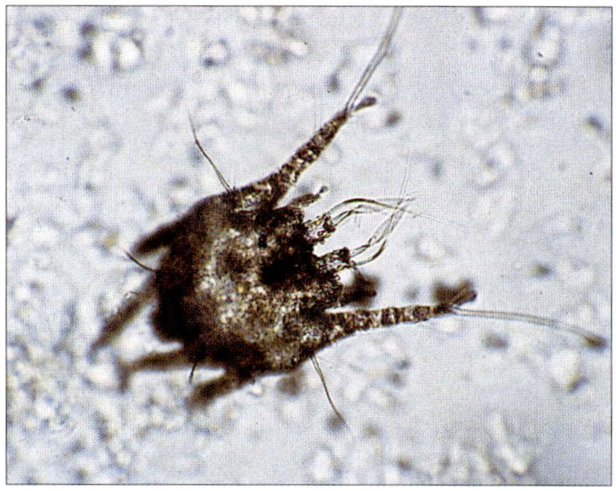

Fig. 111 *A psoroptic mange mite*

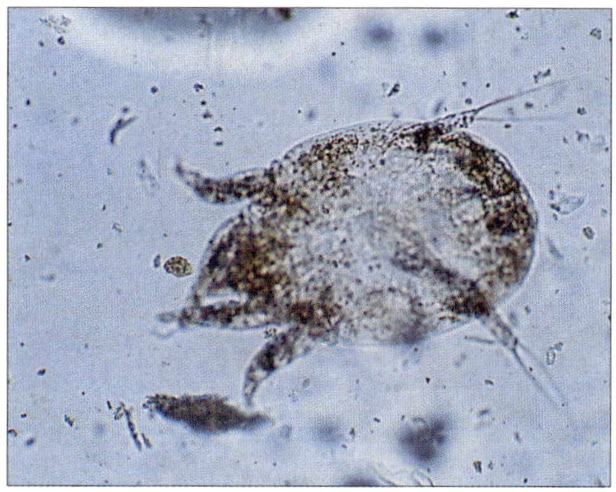

Fig. 112 *A chorioptic mange mite*

Melanoma

Symptoms Rounded lumps underneath the skin, especially in grey horses *(Fig. 113)*. The commonest sites are underneath the tail and around the anus. They can occur internally. Usually, more than one tumour is present.

Cause Melanomas are tumours of the cells which produce the pigment melanin.

Treatment Surgical removal is possible if an individual tumour is causing a specific problem.

Prognosis In most cases good, although the tumours persist. Occasionally they involve a vital structure.

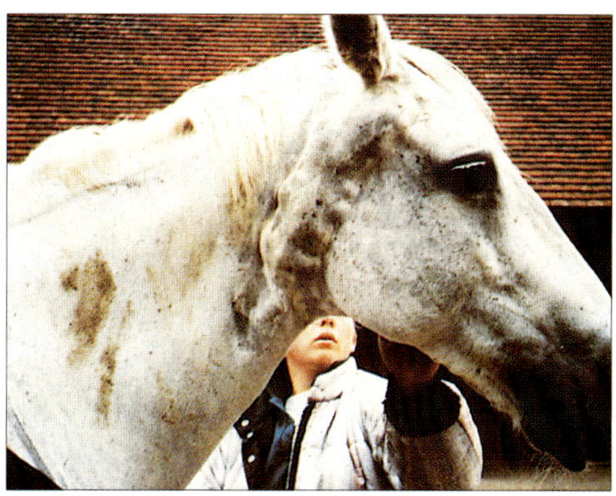

Fig. 113 Melanomas around a horse's throat.

Mud fever

Symptoms Oozing cracks on a horse's heels are often the first sign of mud fever, and may wrongly be mistaken for infected cuts *(Fig. 114)*. As the infection spreads up the legs areas of matted hair develop, held together by thick crusts. The leg may become swollen and this may make the horse lame. Areas with white hair are much more susceptible to the infection than areas with dark hair *(Fig. 115)*.

Cause Dermatophilus congolensis, the organism which also causes rain scald or a staphylococcus. The name 'mud fever' comes from the fact that the infection is often associated with muddy conditions which soften the surface layers of the skin and allow the infection to gain entry. Cold also reduces the surface resistance to infection. The infection is not, however, restricted to the winter months. During warm weather, the abrasive action of dust can similarly allow entry of the bacteria.

Treatment The affected areas must be kept completely dry, and every single crust removed even though this might expose raw skin. The scabs are infective, so they must be disposed of carefully. If a shampoo is used to soften the scabs, a hair dryer or plentiful supply of towels will be needed to thoroughly dry the skin afterwards. There are many antibiotics which will kill the infection once it is no longer protected by crusts. They are applied as a cream every day after the removal of the scabs. If the leg is swollen, systemic antibiotics will need to be given either by injection or in the feed. Oily ointments may act as a protective waterproofing layer during exercise, but should be removed afterwards. They should never be used until all the infection is killed off, or they will seal infection in and protect it just as well as crusts. Non-oily waterproof barrier creams manufactured for human use are even more effective.

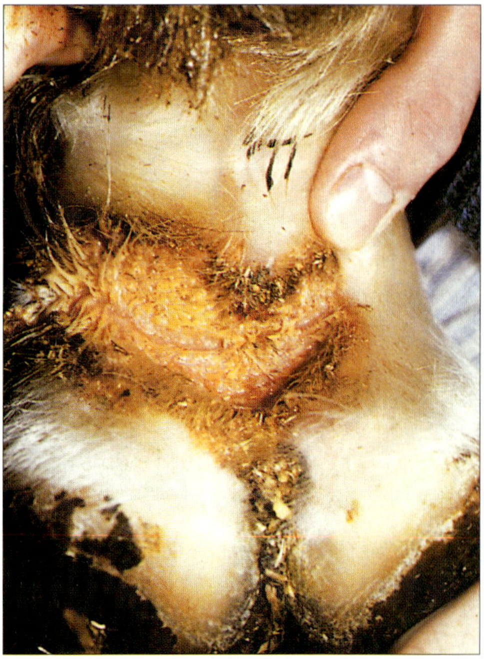

Fig. 114 *Mud fever*
Note the horizontal oozing crack above the heel.

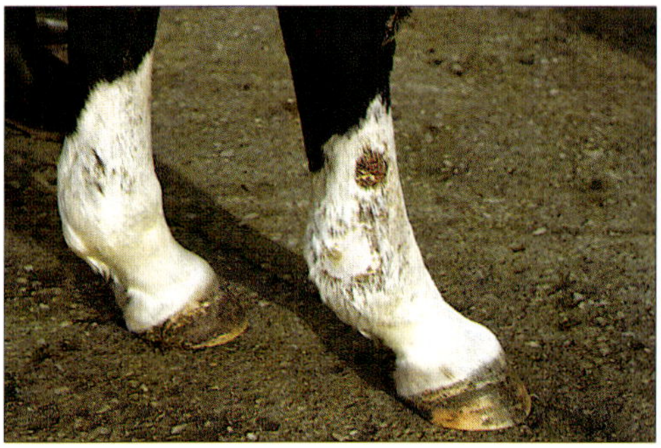

Fig. 115 *Mud fever on the fetlock*

Prognosis As long as all the infection and crusts are removed, it should be possible to prevent recurrence.

Nodular collagenolytic granuloma

Symptoms One or more firm nodules appear in the horse's skin, usually on the back (especially the saddle area) or neck. The nodules are not painful or hot, and remain covered with hair. If the top does become rubbed off, for example by saddle pressure, a hard core, rather like a large grain of sand, may be felt inside the lump. The nodules usually appear during the warmer times of the year. They do not always remain a constant size.They can increase and then decrease in size and may even disappear for a time.

Cause Not known. Under the microscope they look to be an acute localising allergic reaction of some kind.

Treatment May not be necessary because the nodules cause so little trouble. Cortisone injections into the affected area will usually cause the nodules to disappear, but they may return. Laser treatment uses stimulation of natural cortisol levels to do the same thing. Surgical removal of the nodule may be a final resort.

Prognosis Untreated nodules may persist for several years. Even after treatment, more nodules may appear either in the original places or in new areas.

Onchocerciasis

Symptoms Skin irritations, which can be very marked. The commonest area affected is underneath the abdomen, around the umbilical area, but other parts, such as the forehead, can be affected. The affected areas lose their hair, and may become ulcerated. The condition is commonest in older horses.

Cause Onchocerca cervicalis, a parasite worm. Although the adult worms live in the ligaments of the neck, immature worms, called microfilariae, move to the skin. It is these microfilariae which cause the symptoms. The worm is much more common than the skin problem.

Treatment Ivermectin kills both the adults and the microfilariae. Occasionally a reaction occurs around the affected areas as the microfilariae are killed off. Because the parasite is spread by flies, general fly control measures help to limit the problem. Fly repellents should be applied to the horse, and should also be used in the stable if appropriate.

Prognosis Good.

Photosensitisation

Symptoms The white, unpigmented, areas of skin become very pink and inflamed following exposure to bright sunlight *(Fig. 116)*. Blistering of the skin surface occurs. Pigmented areas of the body are not usually affected.

Cause Photosensitisation may arise in two ways. Primary, or direct, photosensitisation is due solely to a reaction to sunlight. Secondary photosensitisation is due to liver damage limiting the breakdown of substances which can react with sunlight. This liver damage can arise from the horse's ingestion of certain poisonous plants.

Treatment Horses must be kept stabled at

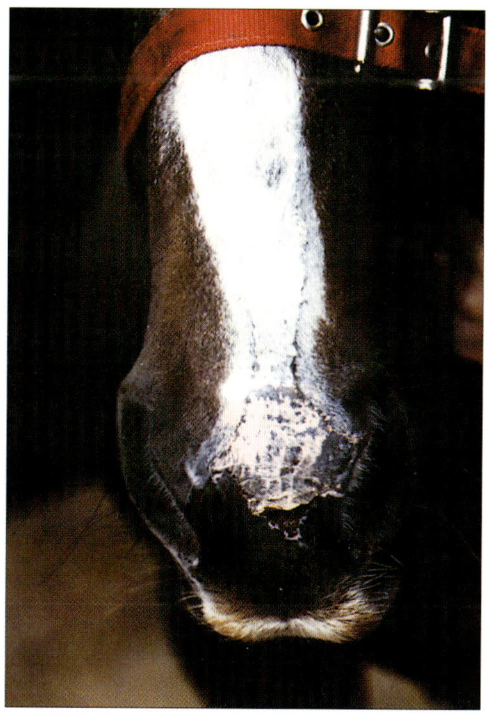

Fig. 116 *Photosensitisation*
Note the cracked skin around the muzzle.

all times so that there is no exposure to sunlight. This also has the advantage of removing the horse from pasture which may contain the poisonous plants. Cortisone preparations, given both by injection and as topical creams, reduce the inflammation. When the horse is not stabled, human sun-screen creams should be applied to the affected areas.

Prognosis The prognosis is good following removal of the underlying cause. However the condition may recur in future years if it is due to liver damage.

Rain scald

Symptoms Small tufts of matted hair appear on the horse's body, especially on those areas where rain might 'run off' the body *(Fig. 117)*. They may appear quite suddenly in warm humid conditions after rain. The tufts are held together by a crust on the surface of the skin and the texture has been likened to a child's paint brush. Unpigmented (white-haired) areas are more susceptible.

Cause Dermatophilus congolensis, which has similarities to both bacteria and fungi. The organism multiplies very rapidly in warm moist conditions and penetrates every microscopic graze and wound.

Treatment The horse must be kept stabled and dry at all times. All the crusts must be removed because the *Dermatophilus* can survive between these crusts and the raw skin underneath, and remain immune to treatment. Once exposed in this way to the lethal effect of drying, most antibiotics and antiseptics will kill the infection.

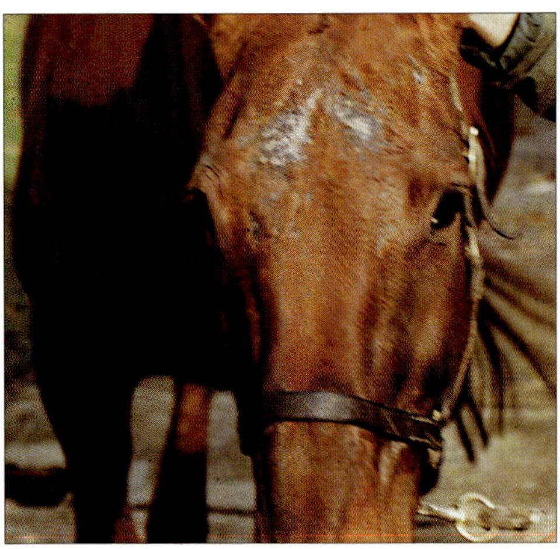

Fig. 117 *Rain scald on a horse's forehead*

Prognosis Some horse are particularly susceptible to re-infection due to a low resistance and/or the presence of much unpigmented skin. Recurrence may be due to a failure to remove and destroy all the crusts.

Ringworm

Symptoms As its name suggests, the classic symptom of ringworm is a circular area where the hair has been lost *(Fig. 118)*. There may be only one or two such areas, or there may be large numbers of them all over the body. Unfortunately, in many cases the affected areas of skin are not circular, and this can lead to problems in making an instant diagnosis. The skin may or may not become crusty and scaly. One useful point is that although the affected areas are often in places which are rubbed by tack, they do not appear to cause any irritation. Also, it may take several months for an infected horse to start showing any symptoms. Ringworm is an infectious disease, so often more than one horse in the yard will be affected.

Cause Ringworm is not a worm but a fungal disease affecting both the top layers of skin and the base of the hairs (the bald areas are due to the weakened hairs breaking off at skin level). Two main fungi are responsible, Trichophyton and Microsporum *(Fig. 119)*.The fungi can be cultured from hairs and scurf taken from an affected area.

Treatment Contrary to folklore, ringworm is not cured by sunlight or by being out at grass. Over a period of months, horses become immune to the fungi. Certain antibiotics, for example griseofulvin, become concentrated in the skin

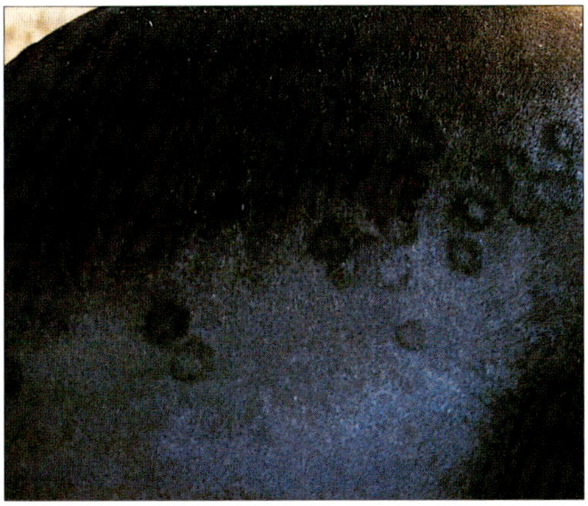

Fig. 118 *Ringworm*
The typical circular lesions can be seen clearly.

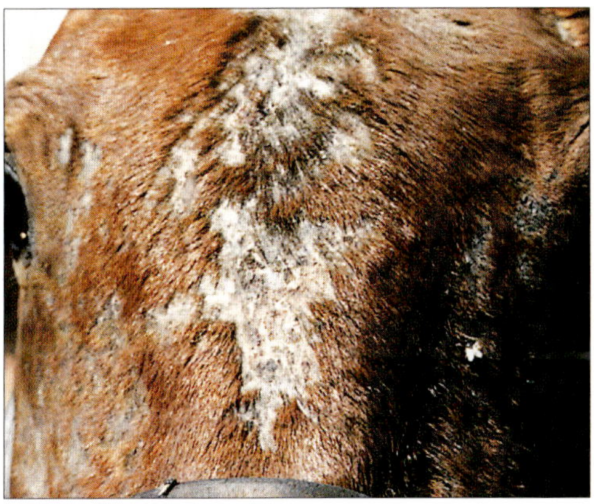

Fig. 119 *Ringworm on a horse's face*
In this case there are no circular lesions.

after being given orally and kill them. Other antibiotics such as natamycin can be used as a wash on the horse and in the stable. Treatment should be accompanied by disinfection of the tack and stable or the horse may become re-infected.

Prognosis As already mentioned, affected horses recover even without treatment. This recovery is slower in horses which are in poor condition. With treatment horses usually make a rapid recovery.

Saddle sores
Symptoms Raw areas of skin appear at places usually covered by tack. The skin becomes markedly thickened and painful.

Cause Friction from badly-fitting tack.

Treatment Obviously the cause of the problem should be removed. Riding should be stopped until the lesion is healed. Surgical spirit is used to 'harden' the skin as long as it is not broken. Malic/benzoic/salycilic acid mixtures speed healing.

Prognosis Good

Sarcoids
Symptoms Large, wart-like tumours appear on the skin of the legs and head, and on the penis. The tumours may become ulcerated and secondarily infected. They are the one of the commonest kinds of tumour in the horse *(Figs. 120 & 121).*

Cause Sarcoids may be caused by a virus similar to that causing warts in cattle.

Treatment Surgical removal can be difficult because they often occur in areas where there is not enough skin left to

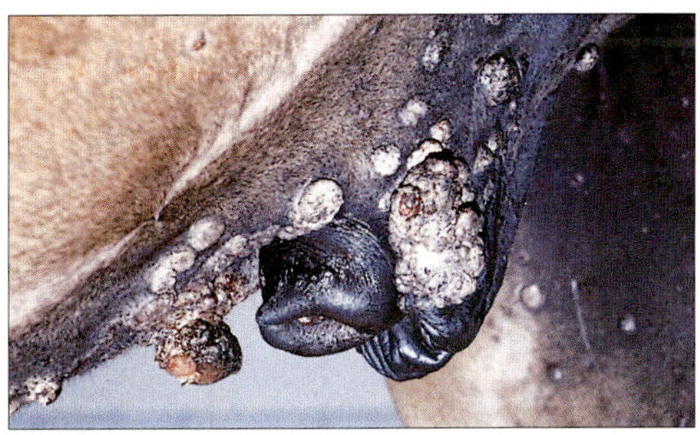

Fig. 120 Sarcoids around a horse's sheath.

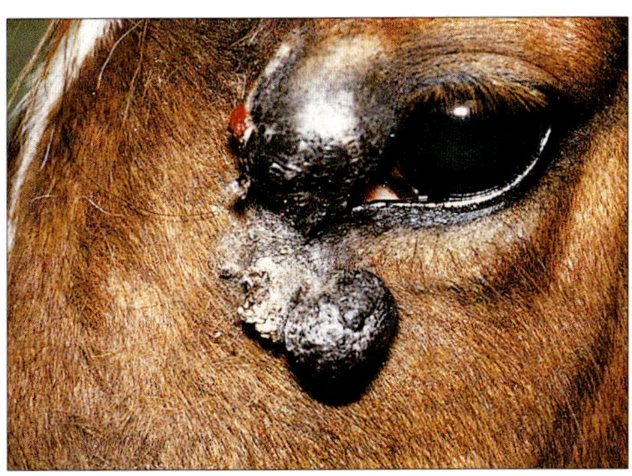

Fig. 121 Sarcoids around a horse's eye.

suture across the incision, and unfortunately they often have no definite 'neck', which can aid their removal. They also occur in areas where there is much skin rubbing, which may lead to wound breakdown. Freezing with cryosurgery and irradiation from radioactive isotopes are used. Injection of BCG vaccine into the sarcoid may, after a marked reaction, cause it to die off. Repeated injections are necessary. These methods of treatment result in an open cavity which takes time to heal.

Prognosis It has been estimated that 50% of sarcoids will reappear after treatment. This is especially likely when the sarcoid occurs in a place where there is a considerable amount of movement.

Scalds

Symptoms An area of moist, acutely inflamed skin is present.

Cause Moist heat such as steam.

Treatment The same as for burns.

Prognosis Generally speaking, relatively small areas are affected by scalding compared with burns. The prognosis is good, although scarring may occur.

Squamous cell carcinoma

Symptoms This is a tumour which affects the skin, especially around the eyes, as well as deeper tissues. Commonest in horses approximately 10 years old. Because sunlight may help to trigger the tumour, it is more common in unpigmented skin. The basic lesion is a nonhealing ulcerated area of skin.

Cause Unknown, although predisposed by solar radiation. It is malignant and spreads to other tissues besides the skin.

Treatment Radiotherapy is increasingly becoming available for horses. Cryosurgery can also be successful.

Prognosis Poor. Even after apparently successful treatment the prognosis is only fair as spread may have already occurred.

Sweet itch

Symptoms The horse rubs its mane and tail against any solid object. The hairs soon break off, and the skin can become very thickened, oozing serum from the raw surface *(Figs. 122 & 123)*. The condition occurs during the summer months, with May and September being the worst times. Even in winter however an affected horse may be spotted because of its short mane and tail. Once a horse becomes affected, symptoms usualy recur every year, often with increasing severity. The older the horse, the more likely it is to be affected.

Cause Hypersensitivity to the saliva of biting midges, particularly Culicoides.

Treatment Corticosteroid injections may relieve the symptoms temporarily, but care should be taken in using this drug in ponies because it may lead to laminitis (see page 76).The only real solution is to prevent the horse being bitten by midges. This may require permanent stabling over the susceptible period with fly netting over all ventilation. Fly repellents may help, both in the stable and on the horse. They require frequent applications, however, and seldom work for more than two to three days. Benzyl benzoate lotion appears to soothe the affected areas and is toxic to the midges. Because the midges are most active during the early and late hours of daylight, grazing should take place either during complete darkness or in the very middle of the day.

Prognosis Affected horses will always be susceptible.

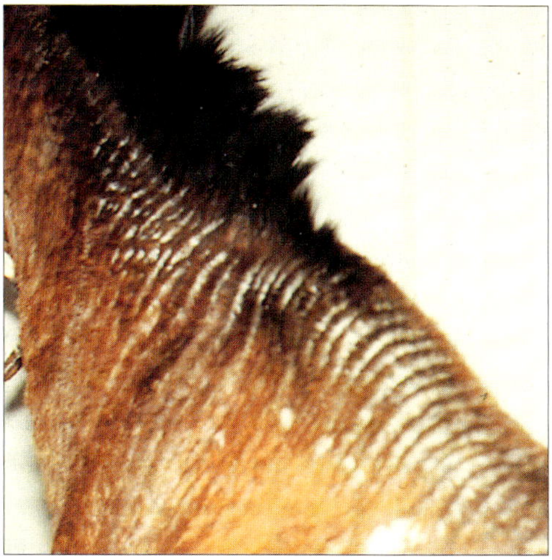

Fig. 122 Sweet itch affecting a horse's mane.

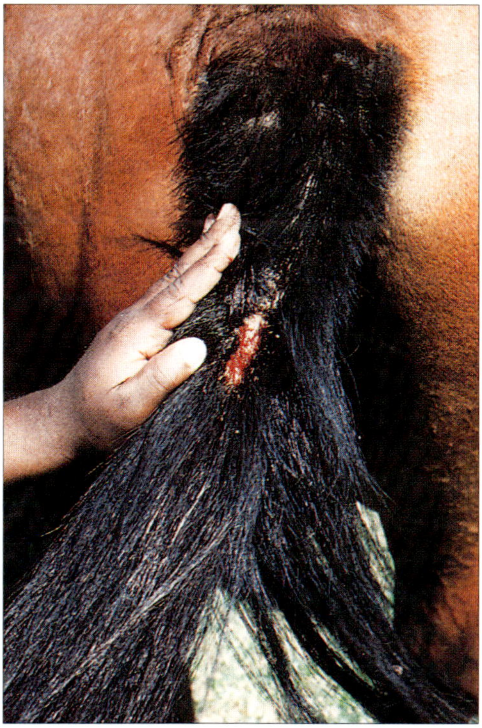

Fig. 123 Sweet itch affecting a horse's tail.

Urticaria

Symptoms Raised areas of oedema appear over the body. When a finger is pressed into these areas, they pit and this depression remains after the finger is removed. The areas of oedema may vary tremendously in number and size. They do not cause any irritation.

Cause Reaction to histamine released as part of an allergic reaction. Obviously there are an enormous number of substances which can be eaten, breathed in or just come in contact with the horse and then trigger off an allergic reaction. Occasionally, veterinary drugs can provide the stimulus for urticaria. Often it is blamed on insect bites, although it is thought that this is nowhere near as common as owners imagine.

Treatment Corticosteroid injections will reduce the reaction. If the problem persists, an effort must be made to discover at least what kind of substance is provoking the urticaria; whether it is occuring in the stable or out at grass. It may occasionally be possible to use a skin prick test to isolate the antigen causing the allergy and then use regular injections of dilute antigen to de-sensitise the horse.

Prognosis The hypersensitivity will persist, so symptoms may recur if the horse comes across the antigen again.

Vitiligo

Symptoms Patches of skin, usually around the eyes or muzzle, lose their pigment and turn pink.

Cause Usually spontaneous, although may be associated with repeated trauma from ill-fitting tack.

Treatment None.

Prognosis Condition permanent but not detrimental.

Warbles

Symptoms A swelling appears under the skin of the back, especially the saddle area, during the spring or early summer. A central hole within the swelling may develop. Once it has appeared, the warble may remain for years.

Cause The warble is the swelling around a larva of the Hypoderma fly. Normally this fly lays its eggs on cattle, but very occasionally may do so on horses. The larvae migrate from the legs, where the eggs are laid, to the back. The hole sometimes seen is the larva's breathing tube. In horses, unlike cattle, warbles may fail to mature and hatch as adult flies. This is why the lumps persist in horses more than they do in cattle. The eradication campaign in cattle has led to its virtual disappearance in horses in the UK.

Treatment Surgical removal of the larva is probably the best form of treatment, although ivermectin will kill it.

Prognosis Good.

Warts

Symptoms The horse may develop literally hundreds of small warts on the head over a short period. They usually have a well-defined 'neck' and they are commonest in young horses. The warts almost always disappear spontaneously.

Cause A wart is a form of tumour. It is benign and does not spread to other parts of the body. Most warts are associated with a virus, which is why several young horses may become affected at once.

Treatment Because the warts disappear when the horse's immunity to the virus becomes strong enough, treatment is not usually necessary. If only a few warts are present, they can be physically removed.

Prognosis As already mentioned, most horses cure themselves in time.

10: Diseases of the heart and circulation

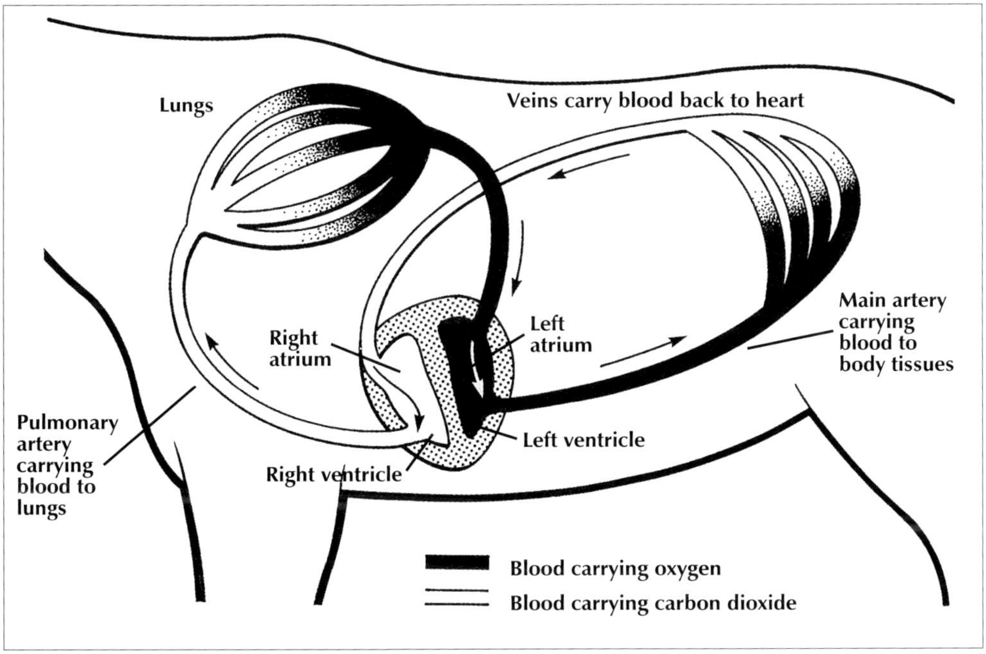

Fig. 124 *The horse's circulatory system*

The way in which the horse's heart and circulation work is much like that of a human. The heart consists of two pumps on the left and right sides *(Fig. 124)*. The right side sends blood to the lungs, which returns, oxygenated, to the left side, from where it is sent around the body. Returning to the right side of the heart, via the veins, it is loaded with carbon dioxide. So, there are two pumps and two circulatory systems, but the heart is common to both.

Blood

Blood is basically water containing, suspended, cells and various chemicals in solution. So, blood is truly thicker than water. By spinning a sample of blood in a centrifuge one can separate the blood cells from the plasma, or fluid. The part of the blood made up of cells is called the packed cell volume (PCV). In a normal resting healthy horse the PCV forms approximately 32–46% of the total volume. If something happens to reduce the horse's fluid levels – e.g. if it becomes dehydrated – the PCV goes up. The number of cells is the same but they rep-

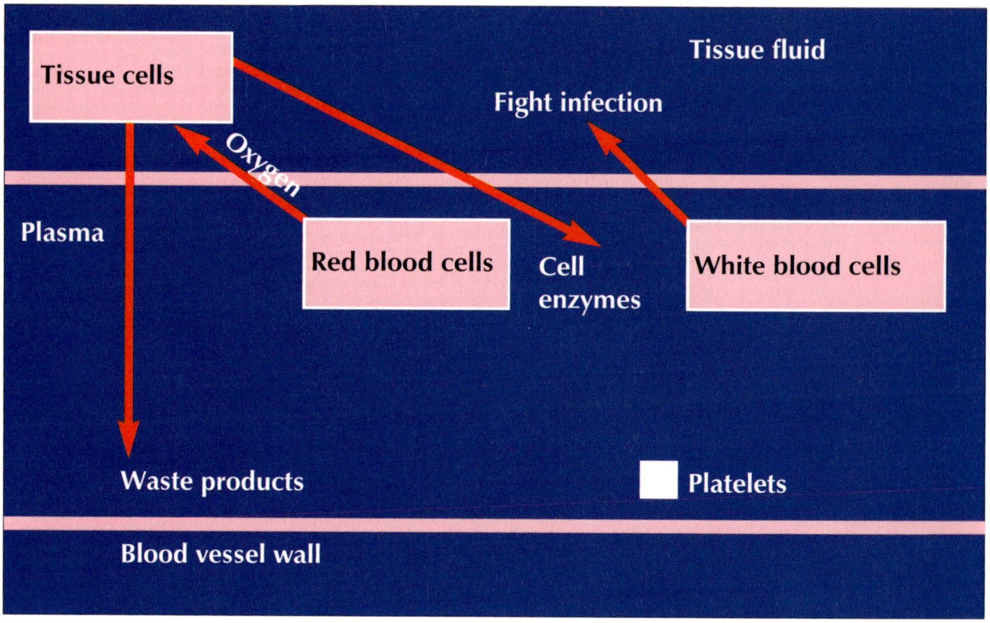

Fig. 125 *The constituents of the blood*

resent a higher percentage of the volume of the blood. If a horse is chronically losing blood, then the PCV may go down because there are less cells.

The fluid plasma circulating around the horse's body is both food supply system and waste disposal system for the body. It contains numerous proteins (around 60g per litre of blood/34.5g per pint), including the globulins, the horse's antibodies to fight disease. The protein level in the circulation determines how much actual water can be transported. If a horse has low blood protein levels, water (or tissue fluid) tends to seep out of the blood vessels into the surrounding tissues. This collection of fluid in the tissues rather than the blood circulation is known as oedema. We can tell if a swelling, perhaps of a tendon, is due to oedema by pressing it firmly with a finger. If the impression remains when we remove the finger, oedema is the cause. If the swelling is due to the accumulation of pus, as in an abscess, the tissues immediately return to their former state when the finger is taken away.

The plasma also carries the 'food' needed by various parts of the body; the glucose, vitamins and minerals without which the muscles or nerves would not function. As already shown, a continuous exchange occurs between the blood and the tissues. The latter absorb their food requirements and at the same time release back into the circulation their waste products for transport to organs such as the kidneys *(Fig. 125)*.

If bacteria multiplying somewhere in the horse's body manufacture bacterial toxins, these will also enter the plasma, to be circulated throughout the body and absorbed by the tissues, with possibly disastrous results. Bacteria and viruses may also enter the cardiovascular system and circulate in the plasma.

When bacteria are circulating in the blood the horse is said to be showing a bacteraemia. When viruses are actively circulating in this way it is a viraemia. It is perhaps worthwhile to distinguish between these two situations and a septicaemia. This term describes a situation where a number of organs throughout the body contain localised foci of infection. For example, salmonella bacteria may initially give a horse diarrhoea, but by the time it dies, they will have established themselves in most of the internal organs, including the lungs, liver, heart etc.

Veterinarians are particularly interested in another group of substances found in the plasma, which are known as enzymes. These are the chemical tools which individual cells use within themselves to perform certain functions. They are kept inside the cell by the cell wall, but a small amount usually leaks out. So there is a low background level of tissue enzymes in the blood all the time, which can be measured. If cells are damaged, more of these enzymes escape into the bloodstream.

An abnormally high plasma enzyme level indicates tissue damage. Often individual organs will have enzymes which are not present elsewhere. So a rise in a particular enzyme level will not only tell the veterinarian that there has been some damage; it could indicate exactly which organ has been damaged and to what extent.

A very good example of this is the use of muscle enzymes in the diagnosis and continuing assessment of azoturia (see page 155). The clinical diagnosis of this muscular condition is confirmed by detecting abnormally high levels of two enzymes, creatine kinase and aspartate aminotransferase, in the blood. In order to prevent further damage to the muscles, the horse must be completely rested until all the muscle damage has been repaired. Blood samples taken during the convalescence period enable the veterinarian both to assess the rate of muscle repair, by seeing how quickly the enzyme levels are going down, and to determine when it is safe for the horse to return to work, by showing that the enzyme levels are back in the normal range.

Plasma also contains various minerals which are vital to the body's normal function. Some of these are present in quite large amounts, such as calcium and sodium, others only minimally, such as selenium—often referred to as 'trace elements'. Food supplement manufacturers stress the levels of trace elements present in their products. It is worth considering that by definition only minimal traces of these particular minerals are needed for the body's vital functions. Seldom does a balanced diet not fulfil these needs. The different tissues of the body require different levels of the various minerals, and it is important that adequate supplies are always available. To achieve this a fixed plasma level has evolved which meets the normal requirements of all the tissues which use each particular mineral.

Although we now know the normal plasma levels of the minerals, this is not quite as useful as it might seem when it comes to diagnosing deficiencies or toxic levels. A very efficient system maintains the plasma levels by drawing on reserves in the body. For example, calcium in the bones is utilised to keep plasma calcium levels constant. By the time this 'topping up' mechanism is exhausted and plasma calcium levels fall, the clinical condition will be so serious that it will already have been noticed. Normal plasma mineral levels should not, therefore, induce a feeling of security. They do not necessarily mean that no problems involving minerals are present in the body.

The blood cells are divided into two groups, the red blood cells (RBC) and the white blood cells (WBC). The red blood cells are so called because they contain a red pigment called haemoglobin. This compound is bright red when it links up with oxygen, but dark red (or even blue) when it is combined with carbon dioxide. Blood leaving the lungs is bright red in colour because it has mixed with oxygen, and all the haemoglobin's 'carrying slots' have been filled with oxygen. When the blood reaches the general tissues of the horse's body, the latter remove the oxygen they want from the haemoglobin. The vacant 'carrying slots' are then filled with carbon dioxide which has been formed in the tissues but which needs to be removed. Blood returning to the lungs has a relatively high carbon dioxide level and low oxygen level. It is dark red in colour. If a horse cannot obtain enough oxygen for its requirements, the haemoglobin (and therefore the blood) can become bluish in colour.

One cannot gauge the haemoglobin levels in the blood from either the appearance of blood seeping from wounds or that taken directly from a vein during blood sampling. Equally, it is not possible to accurately assess the haemoglobin levels by looking at the horse's mucous membranes (the pink membranes around the eyes, inside the mouth, etc.). So-called horse experts tend to look at a horse's gums and pronounce that it looks a bit anaemic, but it has been proved that the haemoglobin levels have to fall to exceedingly low levels before any visible alteration occurs in the mucous membranes. One horse will have different looking membranes from another, but that does not mean that it has different haemoglobin levels. It simply indicates a different concentration of blood capillaries near the surface of the membranes. We use the term anaemia to describe the situation where there is a less than adequate level of haemoglobin circulating in the blood. Anaemia might occur because there is not enough actual haemoglobin available, or because there are not enough red cells present to transport it to where it is needed.

Oxygen transport is one of the most important functions of the blood, and red blood cells far outnumber white blood ones. A healthy horse might have 8–11 x 10^{12} RBC per litre of blood, representing 130 – 170g of haemoglobin, and between 6–12 x 10^{12} WBC. There is also a third type of blood cell—platelets. These are very numerous and are vital for blood clotting—they are usually only counted when a clotting problem is suspected. If insufficient platelets exist, small haemorrhages could occur throughout the body because breaks in the blood cell walls happen continuously even in a normal healthy horse. This is not usually apparent, because the platelet/clotting system seals the haemorrhages almost as quickly as they happen. If there is a platelet deficiency, then these minute haemorrhages, and any major ones, will continue unabated. Boosting platelet numbers by a blood transfusion may stop the haemorrhages.

White blood cells can be of varying types: they were originally differentiated by the shape or character of their cell nuclei. We now know that these visible differences are associated with different roles in the body. Neutrophils *(Fig. 126)* are the cells associated with responses to bacterial infections. They accumulate around the bacteria, and pus largely consists of dead neutrophils and bacteria. Lymphocytes *(Fig. 127)* are the WBCs which manufacture antibodies to fight infection. Eosinophils control the body's sensitivity to foreign substances, so their numbers are increased if there is an allergic reaction or if there are large numbers of parasites present. The largest of the WBCs is the monocyte *(Fig. 128)*. Its numbers often rise if the horse is fighting a viral infection or a long-standing chronic infection.

Much is made of counting the different blood cells in fixed volumes of blood, and using the results both to diagnose what is wrong with a horse and to prognose the outcome. Great care must be taken in interpreting such results because blood is a constantly changing medium. The horse, for example, uses its large spleen like a sponge to store vast numbers of red blood cells. Even the smallest excitement, such as eating hay, causes a degree of contraction of the spleen in order to squeeze some of these RBCs out into the general circulation. This mechanism obviously evolved in order to ensure that if the primitive horse had to gallop away from an enemy it would have enough RBCs to keep its muscles supplied with oxygen.

So, a blood sample taken from a horse at feeding time may appear normal but, in fact, abnormally raised levels have been measured and the resting RBC

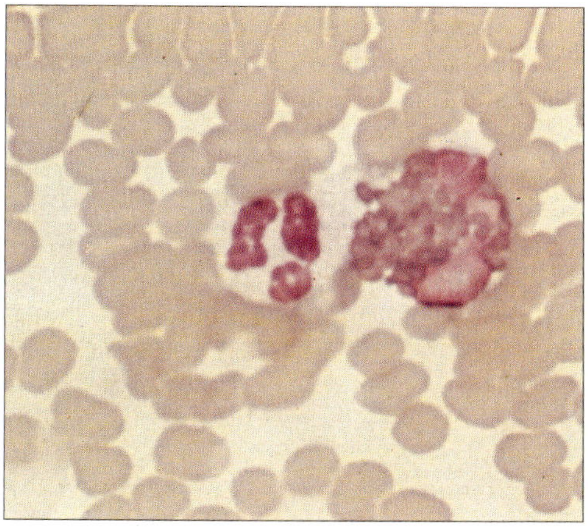

Fig. 126 *Neutrophils*

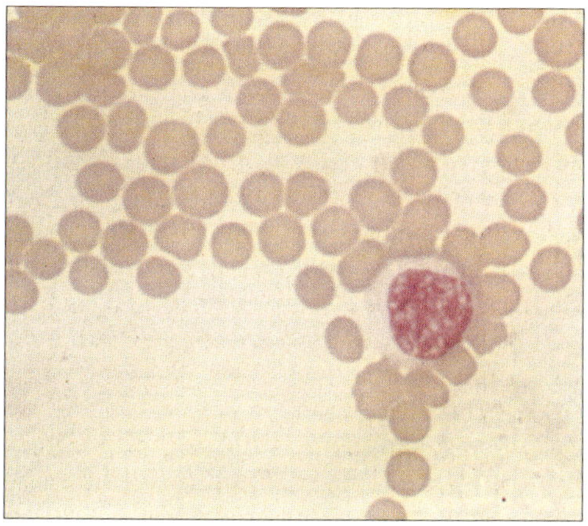

Fig. 127 *A lymphocyte*

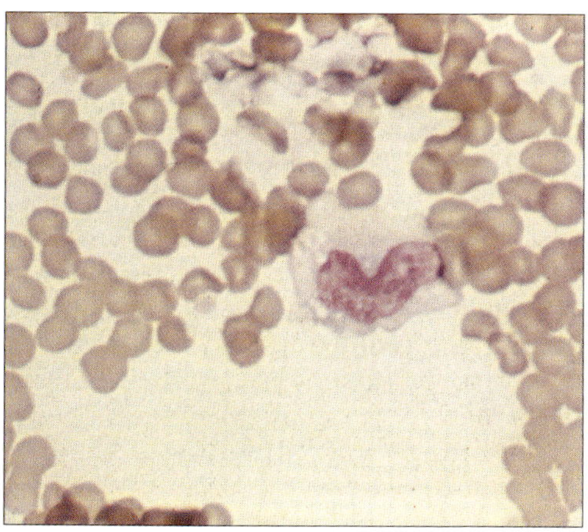

Fig. 128 *A monocyte*

numbers are actually low. On the other hand, a high RBC count in such a horse has no clinical significance, because it is what should be expected in such circumstances. Blood samples should therefore always be taken at the same time of day and in a resting horse if they are to be compared with other results. Although we use average values, you really need to compare results with another sample taken in known circumstances from the same horse if you are to place any degree of reliance on small variations.

Recently it has been suggested that some owners are resorting to 'blood doping' to improve the performance of their racing or competing horses. This technique was developed for human athletes, where the stamina of long distance runners has been improved. Some blood is taken from the horse as it would be if the horse was being used as a blood donor. The blood is carefully stored for four to six weeks, while the horse makes up the blood loss from its body. Just before an important event the stored blood is infused back into the horse, to give it abnormally high levels of red blood cells and haemoglobin. This ensures that its muscles will have plenty of oxygen.

The misguided people who use such illegal techniques do not realise that the horse's spleen already does the same thing quite naturally. No infusion before a competition can increase the circulating RBC numbers as much as can contraction of the spleen, and tests have shown that even with extremes of exercise the horse's spleen is rarely completely emptied of its stored RBCs. Man does not have such a well-developed splenic system, which is why the technique works with human athletes. Whichever species blood doping is indulged in, there is always a health risk. Higher numbers of RBCs increase the viscosity of the blood. It therefore takes more effort to pump the blood around the body, and this can reduce the availability of the oxygen which the technique was designed to increase.

The heart

Although the heart makes up two distinct pumping systems, the two pumps are not identical. The right side of the heart pumps the blood through the adjacent lungs. This requires relatively little physical effort compared to the left side of the heart, which must pump blood to all the other tissues of the body, including the far extremities. As a result the walls of the right side of the heart are much thinner, and the muscles much less developed, than those of the left side. The two sides, though, must each pump a similar volume of blood at each contraction, because the amount of blood which returns from one system provides the amount which enters the pump on the other side.

The actual pumping is also carried out in two stages. The first chamber, the atrium, receives the blood. It is separated by valves from the bottom chamber, the ventricle, which pumps the blood out. The valves prevent blood re-entering the atrium when the ventricle contracts. Again, because of the difference in the amount of force required from the two parts of the pump, the walls of the atrium are relatively thin and weak compared with the walls of the ventricle.

Control of the muscle contractions in the heart is obviously vitally important, and is maintained by the horse in two ways. First, there is the overall control from the autonomic nervous system (see page 53). This ensures that without any effort on the horse's part the heart will keep on beating. Furthermore, the rate and force of those heartbeats will be automatically varied according to the horse's needs. This is achieved by altering the levels of adrenaline circulating in the blood. Adrenaline is a hormone produced by the adrenal gland near the kidney, released into the bloodstream in order to reinstate the heart rate and close down blood vessels supplying non-essential parts of the body. So the heart rate

	Beats /minute
Standing	40
Walking	80
Slow trotting	120
Fast trotting	140
Slow cantering	160
Fast cantering	200
Galloping	225

Fig. 129 How the heart rate is affected by the horse's gait.

automatically increases when the horse is frightened, ready to flee from danger.

We refer to 'the adrenaline flowing' when describing stress. During exercise the muscles need more oxygen, and so the heart rate increases accordingly *(Fig. 129).* But the heart rate of a fit galloping horse is not the same as in an unfit one. Fit muscles produce fewer dangerous waste products and use their oxygen more efficiently, so a fit horse will have a comparatively slower heart rate after a given level of activity. The speed of a horse's breathing and its pulse rate after exercise are not an indication of how much work it has done, but rather of whether the muscles were fit enough to cope with the exercise or whether the heart and lungs had to take the strain. All these factors are automatically weighed up every second of the horse's life.

The individual muscle fibres of the heart must contract at exactly the right time in relation to each other if the blood is to be smoothly and efficiently 'squeezed' from the atrium, through the valves, into the ventricle and then out through a further set of valves. The valves, incidentally, open and close because of differences in the pressure of blood on one side or another. The heart muscles contract as a wave of electrical impulses sweeps across the heart. Although measured in millivolts these

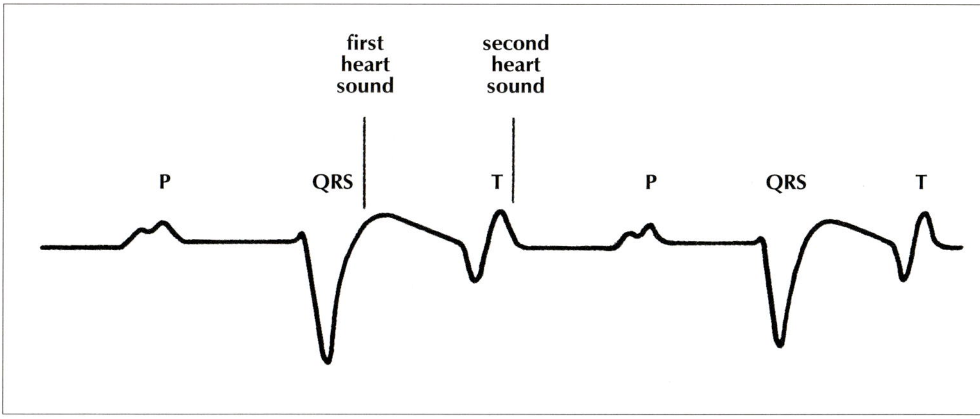

Fig. 130 *An ECG trace.* The wave shows the positive and negative charges sweeping across the heart as they stimulate its muscles to contract.

electrical charges can be picked up at considerable distances from the heart, and they can be displayed as an electrocardiogram (ECG) *(Fig. 130)*. Faults, usually interruptions of the impulses, cause faulty heart rhythms. Heart murmurs, however, are caused by physical abnormalities of the heart valves and the resulting turbulence of the blood passsing through the heart.

We obtain most information about heart function by listening to the horse's chest with a stethoscope. The heart sounds we hear, similar to 'lub dub', are not easy to interpret. There are actually four heart sounds in the healthy horse, two loud ones and two much quieter ones on either side of the main sounds. Additional sounds are usually referred to as heart murmurs, and are relatively easy to hear, though difficult to interpret. Abnormalities of rhythm are hard for the human ear to detect and only the really gross arrhythmias can be appreciated with a stethoscope.

Recently it has become possible to look inside a horse's heart using a machine called an ultrasound sector scanner. This is a development of the scanners used to detect pregnancy in both human beings and horses *(Fig. 131)*. A moving beam of high frequency sound is projected through the part of the body to be examined, and a computer uses the echoes reflected back from the internal structures to build up an image of them. Although not yet widely available, this technique enables the valves of the heart to be examined on a monitor as the heart is actually contracting. This is especially useful in determining the cause, and therefore the significance, of many heart murmurs.

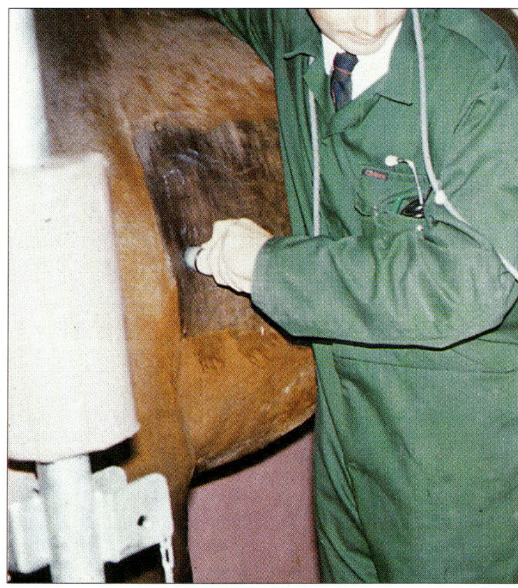

Fig. 131 Using an ultrasound scanner to 'look' inside the heart of a conscious horse.

The circulatory system

The blood is transported around the horse's body via a system of tubes known as blood vessels. Initially, these are large-bore tubes carrying a large volume of blood. They then branch and branch again, like a tree, getting smaller and smaller as the volume of blood passing through them lessens. The arteries have a relatively thick muscular wall in order to maintain the pulsing action of each heartbeat as the blood flows through them. It is this pulsing of the arteries which we note when we 'feel' a horse's pulse. We usually do this where the facial artery passes over the lower border of the horse's jaw bone. If an artery is cut, the blood spurts out forcefully. Depending on which artery is cut it may spurt several yards into the air, due to the great pressure under which it is forced through the arterial system.

When the arteries become very small after many branches, they blend imperceptibly with the next class of blood vessel, the capillary. If the arteries are like the branches and twigs of a tree, the capillaries are the ribs and veins of the leaves. It is from the capillaries that the tissues draw their nourishment. The walls of the other blood vessels are far too thick for any significant amounts to pass through them.

The capillary walls are very thin—often only one or two cell layers thick. Oxygen and other vital substances flow from inside the capillary, where they are at a high concentration, out to the surrounding tissue where they are at a low concentration. Carbon dioxide and waste products, however, are more concentrated in the tissues and so flow down a gradient into the capillaries in order to be transported away. The blood flows quite slowly through the capillaries, under very low pressure. So, capillaries ooze blood when cut rather than spurting like arteries. It is obviously advantageous for the blood to have every opportunity to exchange its various loads as it passes through the muscles and other tissues.

Blood flows back to the heart from the capillaries along veins. These gradually link up with other veins, becoming bigger and bigger as they get nearer the heart. This is the reverse of the route for the arteries but once again the largest blood vessels are nearest the heart. The blood in the veins is at low pressure, being moved along by suction from the pumping heart, so the vein walls do not need to be as thick and muscular as those of the arteries, although they are thicker than the capillary walls.

Interference with blood vessel flow can have various effects. Blocking an artery causes the part of the body supplied by that artery to die due to lack of oxygen and food. Blocking small capillaries has minimal effect because they form such a dense network that there will still be a working capillary somewhere nearby. Blocking a vein results in an accumulation of blood as more and more is pushed out of the capillary bed. The vein becomes stretched by this blood, and eventually fluid starts to escape from the vein through crevices which open up in the vein wall. Note that as the blood cells are too large to escape, fluid passes out into the surrounding tissues as oedema. Some owners' continual bandaging of their horse's legs often leads to swelling from oedema in the unbandaged leg further down. Often this is so slight that it is not observed, and in any case it usually resolves once the bandages are removed and the blood flow can return to normal. It is not, however, a desirable situation for the horse.

No mammal could survive without a mechanism for coping with holes in the blood vessel walls, or it would literally bleed to death. The clotting mechanism is basically the same wherever it occurs, be it artery, capillary or vein. The main difference is that the high pressure of arterial blood washes away clots a great deal more easily than the low-pressure capillary. All blood vessels are lined with a layer of 'non-stick' cells called endothelium. When the blood vessel wall is ruptured the blood cells come into contact with ordinary tissues and possibly air. The blood then clots. A vital part of the clotting mechanism is played by the blood platelets. Platelets and a protein called thrombin act to combine together into a clot which traps other cells and seals the hole in the blood vessel wall. Occasionally something goes wrong and a clot forms inside a blood vessel. It is then called a thrombosis, and may reduce or block the blood flow.

The immune system

As well as the blood circulatory system, there is the lymphatic system. The fluid in this system, lymph, is basically tissue fluid without most of the blood cells (the exception being lymphocytes). The lymphatic system is a drainage system only, draining fluid from the tissues. It incorporates large numbers of lymph nodes scattered around the body. These filter out the bacteria and blood cells present in the tissue fluid when an infection is present. Swollen lymph nodes are often seen when a horse is fighting a bacterial or viral infection. The glands can swell very rapidly if they trap active bacteria or viruses. They do not, however, return quickly to their original, smaller, size when the emergency is over. As a result the lymph nodes around a horse's throat, for example, may stay swollen for weeks or months after the original infection has been overcome. We are usually aware of the lymphatic vessels only when something interferes with general drainage from the horse's hind legs, as in so-called Monday Morning Disease (see page 139), when the thickened vessels can be seen or felt on the inside of the thigh.

Each horse is unique – its cells carry a particular code and there is a unique pattern of proteins in its blood which determines its blood type. Because these proteins are hereditary, passed on from one generation to another, it is possible from a blood sample to confirm or deny the parentage of any given horse as long as both 'prospective' parents have been blood-typed.

The horse's body reacts dramatically with any substance which comes into contact with its blood or lymph not carrying the same 'signature'. Such foreign proteins are called antigens, and the basis of the horse's reaction is the antigen/antibody reaction. Antibodies are neutralising proteins which are formed inside the horse and which combine to make a firm link with any foreign antigens. The perfect antigen/antibody reaction neutralises in an appropriate way any antigen which has entered the body.

Antigens may be merely inert foreign substances, or they may be associated with highly active bacteria and viruses seeking to gain a foothold inside the horse's body *(Fig. 132)*. We can now identify the various proteins, or antigens, within an organ-

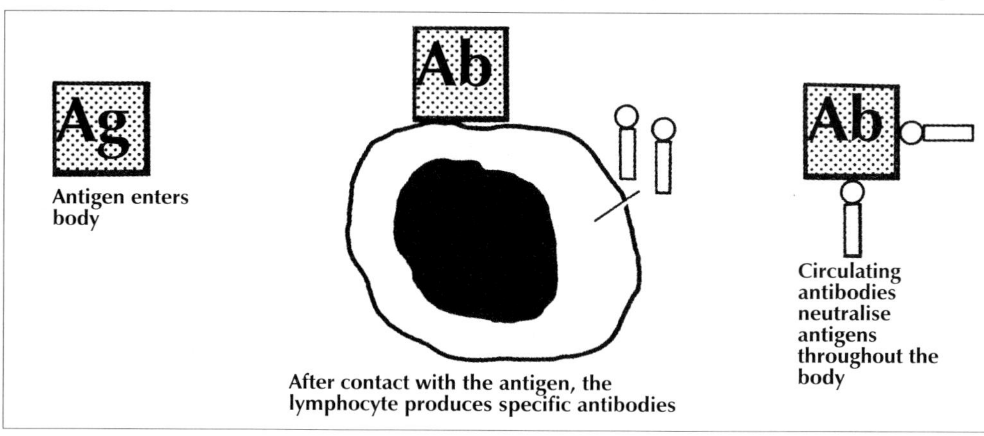

Fig. 132 *The antibody - antigen reaction*

ism such as a virus, and split them up. Using the recently developed techniques of genetic engineering, individual proteins can then be transformed into simple bacteria which can be multiplied rapidly in a laboratory. It does not matter to the horse if the antigen is part of the original virus or a harmless artificially adapted bacterium: it will react to it in the same way with the same antibody reaction because the antibody is specific to the antigen, not to the organism of which the antigen is a part.

Genetic engineering holds out the promise of whole new families of vaccines. Instead of having to culture dangerous organisms in the laboratory, which in the case of viruses is very difficult and expensive, the part of the organism which stimulates immunity is transferred to a bacterium. Once 'captured' in this way, the potentially dangerous part of the organism can be disposed of, and a vaccine manufactured using the adapted, but harmless, bacteria.

Antibodies are produced by lymphocytes and circulate around the body in the blood. Antibodies are not present for an antigen which is making its first contact with the horse. So, a newborn foal has no antibodies at all. The antibodies have to be acquired, either passively or actively. When a foal drinks its mother's colostrum, or first milk, it acquires large amounts of antibodies against all the antigens which have challenged the mare during the recent past. During the first 24 hours of life the foal's intestinal lining will absorb these antibodies into the bloodstream. If the foal drinks enough of its dam's colostrum, it will afterwards have good levels of all the antibodies which were present in its mother's bloodstream. It can therefore neutralise any infections its mother can.

This ability to remain unscathed despite the presence of a foreign substance or infection is called immunity. A foal should be immune to the same diseases as its mother. When we use an antiserum or an antitoxin we are artificially producing the same result. Antibodies against either an infectious organism (in an antiserum) or the toxin it produces (in an antitoxin) are 'harvested' from an immune horse. When they are injected into a susceptible horse they passively make it immune. This immunity only lasts for a few weeks, however, because gradually the antibodies are destroyed and no new ones take their place.

Vaccination

When we vaccinate a horse we hope to provide long-term immunity against an antigen such as a virus, by injecting into the horse's body a safe form of the antigen in order to stimulate the natural active production of antibodies. Usually we use either killed infective organisms or live organisms bred in the laboratory in order to remove their ability to actually cause disease (a process called attenuation). The horse's response is basically similar to both a natural infection and to vaccination. Some of the lymphocytes which come into contact with either the infectious organism or the vaccine particles, make antibodies to neutralise the antigen. Some (called memory lymphocytes) store the information about the antigen in order to enable more rapid and larger scale production of antibodies should the horse ever come across the antigen again.

At least two doses of a dead vaccine should be given. The first one produces a small number of antibodies and some memory cells. These cells respond to the second dose of vaccine and organise the production of a much larger quantity of antibodies. If we use a live vaccine we may only need to give one dose, because the organism lives on in the horse's body and is still present to stimulate the memory cells to produce large quantities of

	Dose needed to stimulate protection	Side effects	Spread to other horses
Live vaccine	Usually only one dose	May actually cause mild disease	Vaccine strain can spread to other horses May revert to disease strain
Dead vaccine	2 - 3 doses	Occasional reaction to adjuvants (chemical carriers) in the vaccine	No effect on other horses

Fig. 133 *A comparison of live and dead vaccines*

antibody. Vaccines do not last forever. In time the memory system fades, and the antibodies wear out. A vaccine cannot offer immunity which lasts for longer than the natural immunity following an infection. In fact, vaccine immunity is often more short-lived than natural immunity. A booster vaccination has to be given before the previous immunity becomes so weak that the memory cells do not respond to the booster.

Live vaccines appear to have an advantage over dead ones, since only one dose is usually required. But there are disadvantages, too. Despite careful selection to eliminate the ability of the vaccine strain to stimulate clinical symptoms, a live organism will always produce *some* reaction in the body. There is also the risk that while it is multiplying in the vaccinated horse, the vaccine organism will revert to its original form and cause full disease symptoms. Sometimes, too, live vaccine organisms spread from one horse to another, so that horse A, whose owner was prepared to accept any side effects, passes the organism to horse B, whose owner was not so inclined *(Fig. 133)*.

If a horse is going to be exported to another country, the country of destination may refuse to admit it if its antibody levels indicate past exposure to a potentially lethal infection. If the horse has been vaccinated with a live vaccine it may be impossible to distinguish between the antibody reaction to the vaccine and that to the infection itself, and entry may well be refused.

Not all infections lend themselves to control by vaccination. Vaccines are most likely to be successful when the immunity stimulated by a natural infection is long-lasting. Immunity following vaccination is never better than that following natural infection, and is often of shorter duration. So, there is a high cost to maintaining this protection, and the owner may forget when booster vaccinations are due. When several strains of the disease organism exist, it may be that the immunity is so specific that infection with one strain does not give immunity against future infection by the other strains. In such circumstances either multiple vaccinations, or the production of a combined vaccine containing all the disease-producing strains, will be necessary. If the disease organism changes its genetic make-up frequently, as is the case with the influenza virus in man, then it may be virtually impossible for the vaccine manufacturers to keep up. This is why influenza vaccination in man has been relatively unsuccessful compared with influenza vaccination in horses, where there are few strains of virus involved which change rarely.

Disease prevention

Although few heart problems can be prevented, many can be limited in their effect. In the majority of cases the circulation is perfectly adequate for low levels of activity, and it is only when the horse is really stressed that insufficient oxygen is circulated to meet the requirements of the muscles and so on. Restricting exercise may therefore be the only treatment needed for a cardiovascular problem. Owners are sometimes concerned that a horse with, for example, a heart murmur may suddenly collapse underneath its rider. In fact surveys show that this is extremely unlikely. When a horse does collapse with a heart condition it is almost always due to the sudden onset of a previously unknown problem. As long as exercise is restricted to that which fails to tire the horse significantly, it should be quite safe.

Some horse owners believe that anaemia can be prevented by spending a fortune on iron supplements.This is not the case. Horses do not commonly suffer from iron deficiency. Nor do they ever suffer from Vitamin B12 deficiency. If production of red blood cells is limited by anything, it is most likely to be a shortage of folic acid, normally obtained from fresh green food.

Dehydration in competition horses can be prevented by ensuring that the horse continues to drink during the actual competition. In the past it was thought that letting a hot horse drink water would cause colic, and so water was deliberately withheld. This practice caused circulatory problems due to dehydration. There is no evidence that drinking water causes colic as long as the horse takes frequent small drinks after the exercise. Horses may need to be 'trained', or encouraged, to do this. They may also need to become accustomed to the taste of the electrolyte solutions which are ideal on these occasions. If suddenly faced with an unusual taste, horses may refuse to drink at the very time when they most need to.

Considering the vital role played by the cardiovascular system in maintaining life, there are surprisingly few specific diseases of the system. Many diseases involve the blood, but only in an incidental way. Most of the problems are self-limiting because they reduce performance and so reduce the demands made upon the system. Of course the antigen/antibody system has a vital role in preventing disease throughout the body. Stress of any kind depresses the immune system, and many of the activities to which we subject horses are associated with stress. We lack a really effective immune stimulant in horses as in all other species. Until one is found, infectious diseases will play a large part in restricting the performance of our competition horses.

African horse sickness

Symptoms Affected horses initially have a fever. The next symptom is often death. In the pulmonary form, coughing and dyspnoea, or difficulty in breathing, follow as a result of fluid collecting in the lungs. In the cardiac form, swellings appear over the body as localised fluid collects under the skin. Heart abnormalities, including murmurs, can be detected.

Cause A virus spread via mosquitoes and biting midges. The disease is almost always limited to Africa, although occasional outbreaks occur elsewhere, most recently in Spain. There are nine different types of virus, each sufficiently different to prevent immunity against one giving protection against another. Vaccines therefore have to cover the particular virus type involved in the outbreak.

Treatment There is no treatment. In affected areas, control of the midges may reduce spread of the virus.

Prognosis 95% of infected horses die. The disease is one of the most dangerous to unprotected horse populations. In the right conditions the virus could wipe out a country's entire horse population, hence the strict international measures to stop its spread.

Anaemia due to blood loss

Symptoms The horse has an increased heart rate. It is dull and has reduced exercise tolerance. Changes in the colour of the mucous membranes will not be visible until the loss of blood is severe. Blood samples reveal the low numbers of red blood cells present.

Cause Haemorrhage is the usual cause. If internal, the owner may be unaware of its existence. Worm infestations can cause chronic blood loss as can some intestinal tumours. Platelet deficiency may result in chronic blood loss.

Treatment Wherever possible the blood loss must be stopped. The volume of blood circulating in the blood vessels must then be raised. It will take at least four weeks for naturally increased production of red blood cells to take effect. Folic acid is more likely to be needed during this time than extra iron. In acute cases transfusions either of blood or chemicals which mimic some of its effects may be necessary.

Prognosis Good in all cases except anaemia due to acute haemorrhage.

Anaemia due to insufficient red blood cell production

Symptoms As this is usually secondary to other diseases, their symptoms may overshadow those of anaemia. The horse has an increased heart rate and reduced performance as it tries to push the same amount of oxygen around the body. It is a chronic disease. Only in later stages will the membranes appear pale, and anaemia cannot be diagnosed merely by examing mucous membranes. Blood samples may show either a low red blood cell count or low levels of haemoglobin in each red blood cell.

Cause Despite the obsession of horse owners, anaemia due to iron deficiency is very rare in horses. It may occur if there is a chronic loss of blood which continually needs replacing. Chronic diseases of many kinds may reduce the number of red blood cells being produced. Lack of folic acid from green food may limit blood cell production.

Treatment Any other problem must first be treated. Folic acid supplements have been shown to increase blood cell production, but large amounts are necessary. Only in rare instances are iron supplements needed.

Prognosis Good except where the bone marrow is damaged by tumours or other disease.

Atrial fibrillation

Symptoms Basically, a lack of exercise tolerance. There may be no other apparent symptom, and the horse may appear completely normal at rest. In more severe cases it may have difficulty in breathing and a jugular pulse (visible pulsations which pass up the jugular vein towards the head). The poor circulation may result in ascites (fluid collecting in the abdomen) or oedema.

Cause Atrial fibrillation is a cardiac arrhythmia. There is an absence of the fourth atrial heart sound. Without the regulating effect of this atrial activity, the heart rate is very irregular. In fact, atrial fibrillation is the easiest heart abnormality to detect on auscultation.

Treatment Quinidine sulphate is the drug most commonly used to treat the condition and restore normal rhythmn. Unfortunately it can produce undesirable side-effects, so a test dose is always given to see whether the horse can tolerate the drug. The side-effects can include further breathing difficulties caused by swelling of the membrane in the nasal passages. The drug acts by slowly controlling the passage of the electrical triggering impulses from the atria to the ventricles. Treatment may need to be maintained for the rest of the horse's life.

Prognosis When atrial fibrillation develops for no apparent reason, most affected horses can be 'stabilised' with medical treatment. If there is also a faulty valve, with a resultant heart murmur, then it is unlikely that the horse will perform normally again. Sometimes the condition occurs in young racehorses during and after a race. Most of these horses will return to normal without treatment.

Babesiosis

Symptoms The horse becomes anaemic, and runs a fever. It develops oedema of the head, legs and lower abdomen. Breathing may be fast. The urine may be discoloured with blood.

Cause A protozoal parasite (babesia) which is spread by ticks in certain parts of the world. Horses raised in these areas often show no symptoms unless severely stressed.

Treatment Ticks must be controlled. Imidocarb will kill the parasite, but there can be side-effects from its use.

Prognosis Good. Treatment is essential to ensure that the horse has not recovered as a symptomless carrier.

Cardiac arrhythmia

Symptoms There may be no symptoms at all. An irregular rhythm may be 'normal' in a horse at rest. It causes concern if it does not disappear with exercise, and serious concern if it is not present at rest but appears with exercise. Exercise intolerance is the likeliest symptom. Many arrhythmias can only be detected by ECG examination.

Cause Arrhythmias are usually due to damage to the fibres in the heart which conduct the impulses controlling heart muscle contractions. Atrial fibrillation is perhaps the most serious 'common' arrhythmia because the atria are contracting rapidly without correlation with the ventricles. Dropped beats occur due to interference in the pathways conducting impulses from the atrium to the ventricle, with the result that at intervals the stimulus fails to get through and the contraction does not take place.

Treatment All treatment must be carefully assessed before requiring the horse to perform strenuous exercise. Quinidine is useful in returning normal rhythm.

Prognosis Dropped beats are normal in many horses. If the arrhythmia is sufficient to cause any clinical symptoms, the prognosis is guarded.

Combined immune-deficiency disease

Symptoms This is a disease of pure or part-bred Arabian foals. The main symptom is lack of ability to fight disease. As the immunity obtained from its dam's colostrum wanes, the foal has a succession of infections until one proves fatal.

Cause An hereditary disease, transmitted by an autosomal recessive gene. Both parents must transmit this gene to the offspring for the condition to occur, and fortunately this happens relatively infrequently. The foal has few lymphocytes (the cells which govern the whole immune process and release antibodies against foreign invaders), even in its lymph glands. It has a poorly developed thymus, which is the special gland present in foals to provide the initial stock of lymphocytes, etc.

Treatment There is no treatment for the condition. Ensuring a good supply of colostrum for the foal may put off the sad day by providing passive protection. Unlike normal foals, however, no active immunity will take over when this wanes.

Prognosis All foals born with this condition die before they are six months old.

Congenital heart defects

Symptoms Often the first symptom is that the foal fails to thrive. It does not grow as fast as expected because of the underlying oxygen deficiency. Sometimes lethargy is the only symptom. If the defect is only minor its effect may not become apparent until the horse starts to be worked, when it shows exercise intolerance. Heart murmurs are detected on auscultation with a stethoscope.

Cause All foals have a patent ductus arteriosus (a so-called hole in the heart) at birth. This usually seals itself within a few days, and only rarely persists in the older foal. The incidence of other defects of embryonic development is low.

Treatment Treatment of such defects is rarely possible.

Prognosis Grave.

Dehydration

Symptoms The horse is weak. When a handful of skin over the neck is pulled up, it stays in a fold rather than immediately becoming flat again. The horse may have a 'thumping' of its diaphragm rather like a hiccup.

Cause Dehydration is not just a loss of fluid; it is also the loss of the electrolytes (or salts) which are dissolved in the body fluid and are essential for activity in all cells. Sodium, potassium, calcium, bicarbonate and chloride are all essential. Both fluid and electrolytes can be lost as a result of diarrhoea. Excessive sweating also causes dehydration.

Treatment Water containing an electrolyte supplement should be available. If the horse has the 'thumps', intravenous calcium is advisable, and intravenous electrolytes may be necessary in any acute dehydration.

Prognosis Good with early treatment.

Endocarditis

Symptoms The horse is dull and lacking in energy or appetite. It may have a high temperature, and the heart rate will certainly be increased. A heart murmur might be heard with a stethoscope.

Cause Most frequently a cluster of bacteria from the bloodstream adhering to the lining of the heart, especially to one of the valves. A blood clot forms around the bacteria causing further interference with blood flow. *Strongylus vulgaris* larvae (see page 81) can end up in the heart with similar results.

Treatment Bacteria can be treated with antibiotics, and worm larvae with a suitable anthelmintic, such as ivermectin. Once the blood clot becomes organised with the formation of fibrous tissue there is permanent damage.

Prognosis Guarded.

Equine viral arteritis

Symptoms The horse has a fever, and pregnant mares may abort. Swellings appear down the legs and around the eyes. The horse becomes weak and may have colic. There is often both a nasal and an ocular discharge. The disease is infectious and spreads rapidly both during mating and by air droplets. Infected stallions often continue to shed viruses in their semen even after apparently recovering clinically.

Cause The cause is a virus infection, which affects the linings of the blood vessels and so allows fluid to 'leak' out into the surrounding tissues.

Treatment There is no specific treatment, but vaccines are now available.

Prognosis Guarded.

Glanders

Symptoms Acute fever. The lymph glands of the head are greatly enlarged. There is a mucopurulent nasal discharge, and coughing. In less acute forms there are nodules in the skin along lymph vessels.

Cause Pseudomonas mallei bacteria. It can also infect carnivores and man.

Treatment Affected horses are usually put down under national control programmes because of the risk to man. The bacteria is sensitive to antibiotics.

Prognosis Poor in the acute form. Some horses recover, or indeed never show clinical symptoms, but still remain infective to other horses.

Haematoma

Symptoms A soft blood-filled swelling under the skin which usually develops quite rapidly and remains the same for several weeks. It is not painful and is not associated with any heart problem or other illness. It can be differentiated from other swellings such as abscesses, by observing whether clear, bloody fluid escapes from a needle inserted into the swelling.

For full details see page 114.

Haemolytic anaemia in foals

Symptoms Affected foals become weak, they may develop jaundice and have blood in their urine. Blood sampling reveals the anaemia. A mare's first foal never gets haemolytic anaemia.

Cause During pregnancy the mare makes antibodies in her blood against antigens from the foal leaking back into her circulation. When the foal suckles the colostrum it absorbs these antibodies from the mare and they destroy its red blood cells.

Treatment The disease can be prevented by denying the foal the mare's colostrum if a blood sample taken during late pregnancy suggests that it will be at risk. The ordinary milk secreted after the first few days of lactation poses no risk to the foal. In severe cases a blood transfusion may be necessary.

Prognosis The condition is fatal without prompt treatment.

Heart attack

Symptoms Horses only rarely collapse from a thrombosis of the coronary arteries. Sudden death during or, more commonly, just after strenuous exercise is often attributed to a heart attack.

Cause Such sudden death is more usually due to rupture of a major internal blood vessel, such as the aorta.

Treatment Death is usually rapid.

Prognosis Grave.

Heart murmurs

Symptoms Often there are no outward symptoms of heart malfunction. Reduced performance may be difficult to evaluate if the owner has no previous performance with which to compare. Heart murmurs are sounds heard in addition to the normal heart sounds. Murmurs occurring during diastole (the time between 'dub' and 'lub') are more significant than those occurring in systole (the time between 'lub' and 'dub'). Murmurs which can be readily heard as soon as the stethoscope is placed on the horse's chest are more significant than those which have to be searched for. Murmurs are often graded on a scale of 1 to 4, and usually only murmurs of grades 3 or 4 cause clinical symptoms. Heart murmurs may only come to light when a horse is examined at the time of sale.

Cause Usually a physical interruption to the blood, causing turbulence. They are often associated with faulty or damaged heart valves. Marked anaemia can cause a murmur due to the altered viscosity of the blood rather than to a permanent physical cause.

Treatment No specific treatment is usually possible, although it may be possible to use drugs such as etamiphylline or members of the digitalis group of compounds to increase cardiac output.

Prognosis Guarded. Heart murmurs are very rarely associated with the sudden collapse or death of the horse.

Heat stroke

Symptoms A body temperature of 106°F (41°C) or higher due to heat absorbed from outside or resulting from heat released during exercise is considered dangerous.

Cause Body temperature is normally controlled at around 101°F (38.5°C) by sweating. As a rule of thumb, if the environmental temperature added to the relative humidity exceeds 180, then heat stroke is likely with any exercise.

Treatment Cooling by water sprays and increasing evaporation with air fans will lower the body temperature to acceptable levels.

Prognosis Good as long as there is no further exercise.

Infectious anaemia

Symptoms The horse has a fever and develops small haemorrhages on the tongue and on the membranes around the eye. This acute stage is usually followed by anaemia, oedema of the legs and possibly jaundice. The horse gradually loses weight.

Cause The disease is caused by a virus, spread by flies. Once infected the horse is infectious for the rest of its life.

Treatment There is no treatment, nor is there an effective vaccine. Movement of horses from areas where the disease occurs is usually restricted.

Prognosis Grave. Euthanasia is often carried out to reduce the danger of other horses becoming infected.

Monday morning disease

Symptoms Oedema of the lower parts of the hind legs is seen following a period of rest on full rations. The fluid accumulates due to leakage from the lymphatic system. The legs are warm and obviously painful when touched. The lymph glands in the horse's groin may also be hot, swollen and painful.

Cause The cause is a combination of a lack of exercise and high-protein food. Traditionally this occurred in draught horses after their Sunday rest day.

Treatment Gentle exercise and the use of diuretics to reduce the oedema. Prevention consists of always reducing the feed when the level of exercise is reduced.

Prognosis Good, although repeated attacks can permanently damage the walls of the lymphatics.

Potomac horse fever

Symptoms The horse runs a fever and has profuse watery diarrhoea.

Cause A single-celled rickettsial parasite called *Ehrlichia risticii* which lives in the monocyte blood cells. Transfer between horses is by blood-sucking ticks.

Treatment Rickettsia are sensitive to the antibiotic oxytetracycline.

Prognosis Poor. There is a high fatality rate.

Purpura haemorrhagica

Symptoms Oedema develops on the head, limbs and ventral abdomen. Very small haemorrhages develop on the pink mucous membranes of the mouth, eyes etc. Breathing may be difficult because of oedema in the lungs. Symptoms usually appear two to three weeks after an infectious disease such as a Streptococcal infection.

Cause Immune reaction to the infection in the blood vessel linings.

Treatment Corticosteroids may need to be given for two to three weeks. High doses of penicillin are given to kill any remaining streptococci.

Prognosis Guarded.

Shock

Symptoms Shock is the body's attempt to concentrate on its life-support systems only. There is a generalised shutdown of blood vessels, which results in the horse feeling cold and the muscles being very weak. Digestive activity ceases. The heart rate is usually increased, while the circulation remains weak.

Cause Many causes, such as acute infections, laminitis, severe colic etc.

Treatment The blood volume must be increased and the general circulation helped, so large volumes of fluids need to be infused intravenously as soon as possible.

Prognosis Guarded.

Thrombophlebitis

Symptoms Thrombophlebitis is the blocking of a blood vessel by a thrombus, or blood clot. The blocked vein becomes hard and may at first be painful. The part of the body drained by the vein may develop oedema. If the clot which blocks the vein becomes infected, an abscess will develop. Thrombosis of the aorta causes hind leg stiffness which increases during exercise.

Cause Often, reaction at the site of an intravenous injection. Thrombosis may also follow a generalised virus disease such as viral arteritis.

Treatment Anti-inflammatory drugs are used to control the reaction in the wall of the vein. Hot fomentations may give some relief. Antibiotics are needed if there is any sepsis.

Prognosis A collateral blood supply usually develops to supply the part of the body normally supplied by the blocked vein, although this takes time.

11: Movement, lameness and the locomotor system

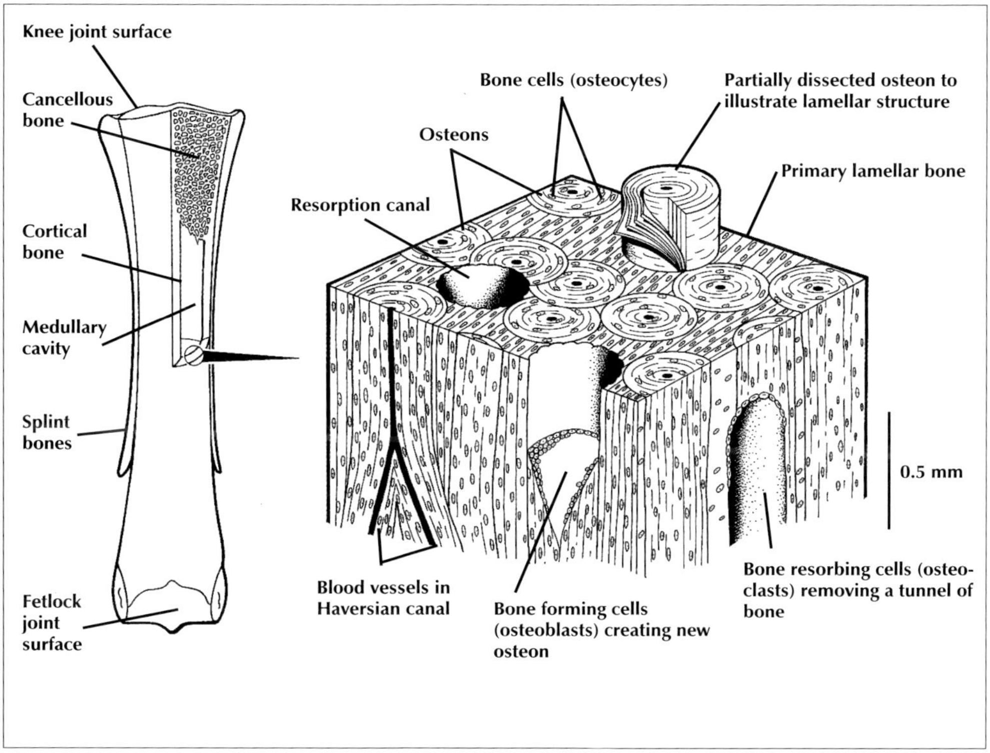

Fig. 134 *The structure of bone*

It is important to appreciate the size and complexity of the musculoskeletal system. Although it has a large number of individual components performing distinct functions, there is a tremendous degree of interaction. This makes it difficult to break the system down into its component parts and descibe them in isolation.

Bone and cartilage

Bone *(Fig. 134)* consists of an organic component, a framework or matrix composed of collagenous fibres, and an inorganic or mineral component, chiefly calcium phosphate and calcium carbonate, whose crystals are laid down by cells called osteoblasts. Each bone is covered with a 'skin' called the periosteum. The inner layer of the periosteum contains osteoblasts, or bone-producing cells, increasing the diameter of the bone either locally or along its whole length. The bone substance near the surface and the periosteum is dense, i.e. it has a high concentration of bone crystals and few cavities. This bone is known as cortical bone. Deeper into the bone, the substance is less dense although it still has girders, or trabeculae, of denser bone running through it. This bone is called cancellous bone.

As a rule, we do not naturally think of bone as needing a blood supply in the same way as does the skin or the muscles, but bone is very much a living tissue. If it does not have a proper blood supply, bone dies just like any other part of the body. Any condition which reduces the blood supply to an area of bone is likely to be associated with pain and lameness. The blood circulates through arteries and veins in bone, in what are known as Haversian canals which also contain lymph vessels and nerves. The large long bones, such as the femur, have a cavity along their centre which is called the marrow cavity. It is filled with a spongy mass of blood cells, fat cells and the tissues which manufacture more blood cells.

As a foal grows, so its bones must grow. This is not achieved merely by adding an extra layer around the whole bone, because this would result in extremely thick bones. Instead, the immature bone has special areas called growth plates, or epiphyses. An epiphysis is rather like a disc of bone which lays down new bone on either side and so 'pushes' the end of the bone away from the central shaft. In this way the bone grows in length while its diameter increases more slowly, with maturity. The epiphyses are the most delicate parts of the skeleton. Young bones often break along the line of such a growth plate. Uneven growth at a particular growth plate gives rise to a deformed bone and so faulty conformation. Conversely when a growth plate closes, and stops its activity, no more growth can take place in the length of that bone.

Given the dire consequences of a broken bone, it is worth considering what happens if a fracture occurs. The horse's body reacts by attempting to establish some link between the two separated fragments. It does this by forming fibrous tissue which extends from both fragments until they are joined together. Although such fibrous tissue (which is mainly collagen) may feel hard to the touch, it is not rigid enough to stand the strain of movement. At this stage, therefore, the broken bone has been made safe in that the fragments can probably no longer cause damage to the surrounding blood vessels and muscles, but the horse is still lame and unable to use the bone properly. In some cases this is where the healing process ends, and the horse never regains the full use of the fractured bone. Only if the fibrous tissue becomes ossified (changed to bone) will the bone be able to function normally again, and if there is any significant amount of movement between the two fragments, ossification will not take place.

Proper ossification requires osteoblasts to spread through the fibrous tissue and to start to lay down bone. Eventually, all the fibrous tissue becomes converted into bone, and the periosteum extends over this new bone to complete healing. If the fragments involved in the original fracture were not separated very much from each other, and there was little or no movement between them, the healed fracture will only have a small amount of new bone.

This is the situation we seek to achieve when attempting to mend a fractured bone. If, however, much fibrous tissue had to be formed before the fracture was stabilised enough to heal, then there will be a considerable amount of new bone, or callus. This callus may cause problems of its own, either by surrounding and anchoring adjacent tissues or by interfering with movement at joints. In ideal conditions ossification takes around three weeks, and a healing fracture is healed enough to withstand movement (though not necessarily strong fast move-

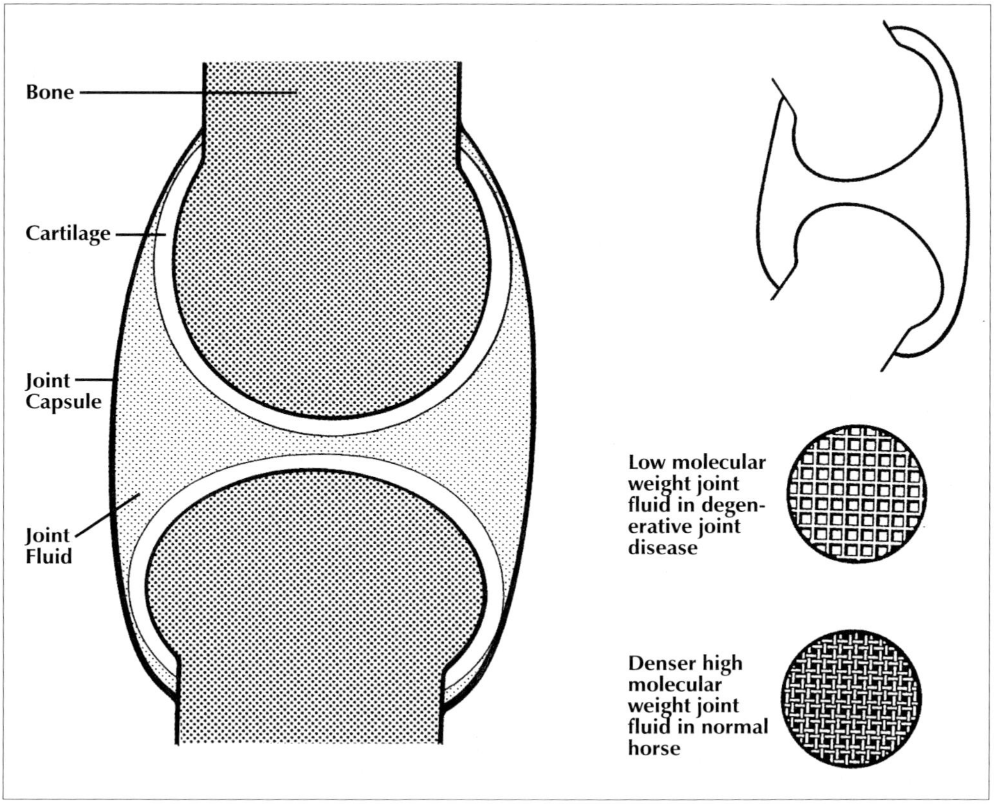

Fig. 135 *Joints and degenerative joint diseases*

ment) after six weeks.

A joint is the arrangement used to enable one bone to move against another *(Fig. 135)*. This specialisation is necessary because if one bone rubbed against another, the friction caused would soon wear them away. Therefore, surfaces of any two adjacent bones which might possibly come into contact with each other are covered by cartilage. This can be thought of as a softer form of bone which has an abundant intercellular substance that gives it a firm consistency well adapted to permit smooth gliding movements between the opposing surfaces. Even so, some form of lubrication is needed to try to ensure that movement, thousands of times per day, 365 days a year for many years, does not wear through the cartilage. This lubrication is provided by a special joint (synovial) fluid.

The joint fluid also supplies the cartilage with nutrients. It is mostly made up of molecules of a substance called hyaluronic acid. The basic molecules of this acid are relatively short, but in joint fluid they are polymerised, or joined together, to make very long molecules which mesh together. This meshing gives joint fluid its thick consistency, and its remarkable anti-friction properties. When a joint is damaged the polymers may be broken down by the inflammatory reaction, with the result that the hyaluronic acid molecules are shorter and do not mesh together so well. So, just when the damaged joint needs the most lubrication and cushioning effects, the joint fluid is unable to provide them. Even after the initial inflammation subsides, low molecular weight hyaluronic acid may continue to be released into the joint. As a result lameness may persist.

Interestingly enough, replacement of such low molecular weight hyaluronic acid by the high molecular weight material (either from a healthy joint of the same horse or by an artificial product) may stimulate the production of normal joint fluid. As a result the horse may become sound again. Naturally some sort of barrier is needed to contain the joint fluid, and this is provided by the joint capsule which is attached to the bones and seals the joint. The capsule is lined with a synovial membrane which secretes the joint, or synovial, fluid.

In most cases the joint capsule is not strong enough to stabilise the joint and prevent the bones involved from being pulled away from each other. Some joints, such as the hip joint, use a ball and socket arrangement to provide stability through a wide range of movements. Others, such as the knee joints, are more like hinges without a physical link at the hinge. In these joints particularly, a strong system of collateral ligaments is needed to give stability.

Ligaments and tendons

There is some confusion over the difference between a ligament and a tendon, and there are those who are unaware of any difference at all. A ligament joins two bones, so providing stability during movement, but not generating the movement itself. A tendon, on the other hand, links a muscle to a bone (almost every muscle ends in what is termed a tendon of insertion), and is involved in initiating movement. But ligaments only respond passively to involvement in movement.

This difference in function is reflected in their main structural differences. Ligaments have a relatively high percentage of elastic fibres so that they can stretch slightly during movement and then 'pull' the bones back to the resting position. Tendons have a relatively high percentage of collagen fibres in order to pass on almost all the pull from the muscle to the bone. Collagen is a very strong protein, well suited to the tendon's role of transferring the force of the muscle contraction to the bone. In tendons, most of the collagen is present as collagen type 2. The molecules are arranged in a crimp (or zig-zag) formation which allows a certain amount of extension (straightening out the crimp pattern) but within very precise limits. When that limit is reached, fibres must tear to allow the tendon as a whole to give.

Most tendons are very short, but this is not possible in the horse's lower limbs, where the muscles are separated by a considerable distance from the bones they have to move. There are no muscles below the knee or the hock, and yet these joints may be 45cm (18in) from the pedal bone. A long tendon is not necessarily weaker than a short one per unit length, but there is more chance of it being injured. The force exerted on the flexor tendons of the horse's leg at the gallop has been estimated to be around 22–33,000N units. As tendon tissue is only capable of withstanding a force of 25–50,000N units, it is perhaps not surprising that injuries should occur, because at speed the horse is always operating in the danger zone.

When tendon fibres are over-extended and torn, the small blood vessels which lie between them rupture and a blood clot forms, permeating the inflamed region. The blood supply to the central area of a superficial flexor tendon down the back of the cannon is not as great as that to a muscle, but it is sufficient to ensure that a blood clot instantly forms in the injured tendon. This clot becomes organised into granulation tissue, which is the body's all-purpose healing tissue. The granulation tissue contains many anti-inflammatory cells, new blood vessels and type 1 collagen fibres. Unfortunately the collagen fibres within the tissue are randomly arranged, not at all like the orderly pattern described earlier which is needed for maximum strength. With the passage of time, there is a tendency for the granulation tissue to become less cellular, and for the collagen fibres to become more regularly aligned along the direction of normal pull. At the same time the collagen changes from the type 1 form which is originally formed to the stronger type 2 collagen.

A healed section of tendon can become, in time, as strong as the original it replaced. It must be remembered, however, that it never completely regains its original structure, so there are slightly weaker areas where normal and abnormal tissue blend into each other. Also, as a result of either the extra weight it has to bear or to some message sent from the injured leg, changes occur on the corresponding tendon of the opposite leg during the convalescent period after a tendon injury. Although these changes may not be detectable clinically, they do occur, and mimic some of the changes in collagen structure that occur with injury (weakening it accordingly). This is why so many horses sprain a tendon in the other leg after the initial injury appears to have healed.

Tendons move physically as the bones respond to their tension. In order to reduce friction along the whole length of the tendons they are encased within a sheath, rather like the insulation around a wire. There is a tendon fluid lubricant bathing the tendon and helping it to move freely within the sheath. The walls of a tendon sheath are not very thick, and often the first time a horse owner becomes aware of their existence is when the sheath becomes swollen by extra fluid as part of the inflammatory response to an injury. One of the dangers associated with inflammation of a tendon sheath is that strands of fibrin can be formed in the inflammatory fluid and these limit normal movement of the tendons and sheath, i.e. they form adhesions. The longer the tendon sheath is swollen and inflamed, the more chance there is of adhesions forming. Conversely, the sooner we can reduce inflammation, even if the necessary treatment is either time-consuming or expensive, the less chance there is of adhesions permanently affecting movement either clinically or subclinically.

Tendon sheaths have little tolerance to infection. If an infection penetrates the sheath, there is an immediate and dramatic response. The horse can, within an hour or two, become so lame that it cannot put the leg to the ground. Indeed, the pain may be so great that it looks as if a bone has been broken.

Another situation where the tendon/tendon sheath system might be said to over-react is when excessive pressure is applied, for example by a tight bandage. The resulting disturbance of fluid and blood circulation causes similar symptoms to those seen with a sprained tendon, and is just as difficult to deal with. The moral is: 'If in doubt, do not bandage a horse's tendons'.

Muscles

I mentioned earlier that tendons provide the link between muscle and bone (page 144). The muscles provide the whole range of movement which occurs in the body from one simple action/contraction. Two systems are needed for each movement; one pulling in one direction when it contracts, and the other pulling in the opposite direction while the first system relaxes. This applies both to the muscles we can see articulating the skeleton, the head and so on, and to the muscles in the walls of tubes such as blood vessels or airways. Because of their appearance under the microscope, muscles of movement are sometimes referred to as striated muscle, and mus-

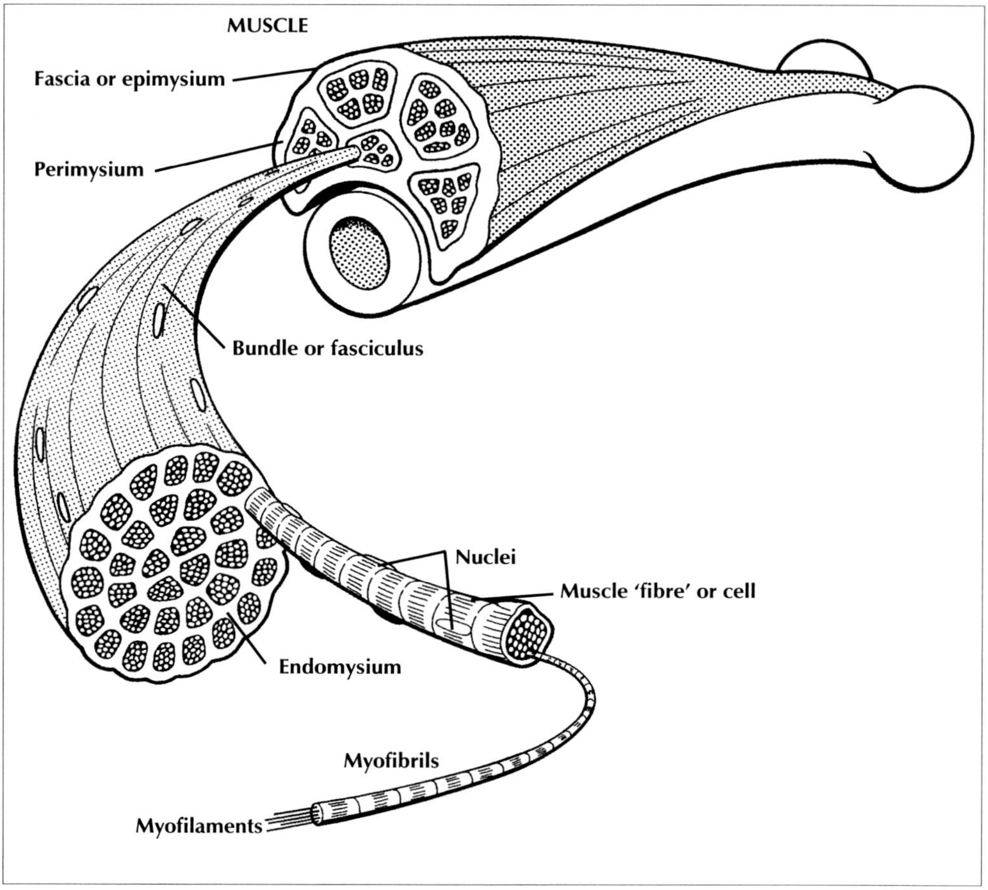

Fig. 136 *The microscopic structure of muscle*

cles in blood vessels are referred to as smooth muscle.

The two systems need not be of the same strength. It takes considerable strength to pull a leg backwards when it actively propels a horse forward, because the horse's weight is also being supported. It takes much less effort to place the same leg forward ready for the next stride because the leg at that precise moment is not bearing any weight. So the muscles associated with pulling the leg backwards (the flexors) are always particularly well developed, while those associated with placing the leg forwards (the extensors) are smaller and weaker. An injury to a flexor will therefore have more far-reaching consequences than an injury to an extensor.

Structure of the muscle

Each muscle consists of many bundles of muscle fibres *(Fig. 136)*. The bundles are held together by fibrous connective tissue, which naturally has to be quite strong to cope with the strong physical forces involved. An extensive network of blood vessels connects the individual fibres (which is why whenever a muscle is cut it bleeds so profusely). There is also a sensory network of stretch receptors, which monitor the state of the muscle and return the information to the central nervous system, since it is vitally important that contraction of the muscle is properly coordinated. If it were not, the bundles of fibres would literally tear themselves apart. This is precisely what happens when a tired horse suddenly goes lame as a result of a 'pulled muscle'. The contractions become uncoordinated and damage themselves rather than being damaged by external forces.

Each muscle cell, or fibre, has not just one but many nuclei. This is because the length and mass of each cell is the result of the fusion of more than 100 cells. Within each muscle fibre there are many rod-like fibres of proteins called myofibrils. Each myofibril in its turn contains myofilaments of two proteins called actin and myosin. There are chemical bridges which hold the actin and myosin filaments interdigitated with one another. When contraction occurs, changes in the chemical bridges slide the filaments even further in between each other. The distance the individual filaments move is very small, but when magnified by the numbers present it can produce a dramatic shortening of the muscle, and initiate movement.

The harder a muscle fibre works, the thicker it becomes. So, a horse in full training has basically the same number of muscle fibres as it does when roughed off in a field. The difference in size of each muscle is due to greater individual muscle fibre mass rather than increased numbers of muscle fibres.

Providing the muscle with energy

When we run, we stimulate muscle activity which requires energy. This energy production requires adequate supplies of the basic ingredients fuelling the process. The changes in chemical bridging which result in contraction can only occur if energy is available. When the energy supplies are exhausted, no further muscular contractions are possible. The key to energy production is a compound present in all cells, called adenosine triphoshate, or ATP. In the presence of a special catalyst, or enzyme, ATP can combine with water to form adenosine diphosphate (ADP), phosphate (P) and energy:

$$ATP + H_20 \longrightarrow ADP + P + Energy$$

Only about 25% of the energy released by this reaction is actually mechanical energy used for the muscle contraction, so it is not a terribly efficient system from one point of view. The rest of the energy released is in the form of heat, which is why a horse gets hot when it gallops. However, the system is very flexible because the whole process can be reversed, so that:

$$ADP + P + Energy \longrightarrow ATP + H_20$$

The rate at which the ATP is reformed must equal the rate at which it is broken down, or again muscle contraction will stop. The faster the horse moves, the faster the replacement will need to be. The energy needed to replace ATP comes from the 'burning' of food, especially carbohydrates and fats. Such burning of fuel to provide energy is dependent on the presence of oxygen and is described as aerobic energy production.

When oxygen supplies have been exhausted during strenuous exercise, carbohydrate in the form of glucose can still produce energy. The glucose is broken down into lactate (or lactic acid) and ATP. The lactate is toxic to the muscle cells if it accumulates in any quantity, and muscle contraction can then no longer occur. Energy production involving lactate production is said to be anaerobic. For safe and plentiful energy production, and thus maximum muscle contraction, the horse needs to produce as much energy aerobically as possible. The main effect of training is to increase the amount of aerobic production compared with the amount of anaerobic production. One of the main aims of nutrition is to ensure an adequate supply of glucose and other fuels to satisfy energy demands without needing to draw too heavily on reserves, some of which may only be able to release energy anaerobically anyway. Fatigue, or tiredness, is the failure of muscles to contract fully because of the build-up of lactate during anaerobic energy production. It is, of course, a temporary state. Given enough time and fuel, the muscles will eliminate the lactate and restore the ATP levels.

Structure of the legs

The horse is a four-legged animal, but it does not divide its weight equally between the four legs. The front legs bear approximately 60% of the weight, compared with 40% on the hind legs *(Figs 137 & 138).* This is one of the reasons why lameness is more common in the front legs than the hind legs. The weight of the heart, lungs and abdominal organs can be considered to be suspended from the spine rather like a suspension bridge, with the legs acting as supports at each end. The weight of the horse's head presents a problem. Despite the weight-reducing effect of the large air-filled sinuses in the skull, it is still very heavy, as anyone who has tried to support a horse's head will confirm. This is because it is used as a balancing organ. With the weight of the head in front of the forelegs, using the neck as a lever particularly balances the weight of the hind legs. This effect is most important when the horse jumps. The head going over the jump pulls up the hind legs even though the fulcrum, the forelegs, is off the ground. A failure of balancing equilibrium on landing ends in disaster with the horse collapsed on the ground. Powerful muscles and ligaments have evolved in the horse's neck to support the head and control its movement for balance.

The front legs do not have a bony connection with the rest of the skeleton. In man, the collar bone fulfills this function, but in the horse the forelegs are only connected to the rest of the body by muscles which attach to the ribs and spine. It might be considered that this is poor

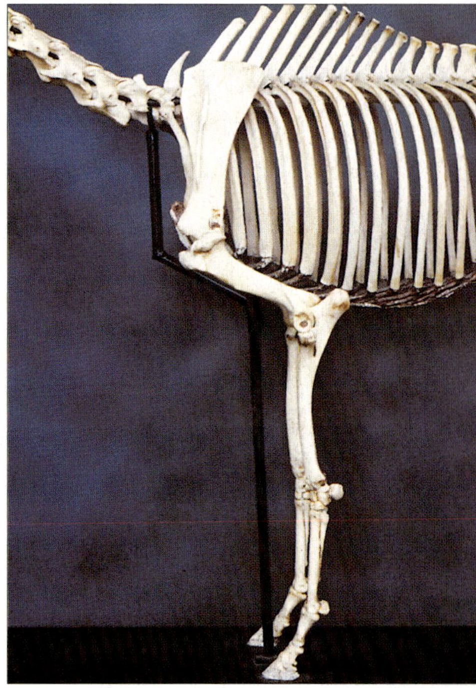

Fig. 137 *The foreleg skeleton*

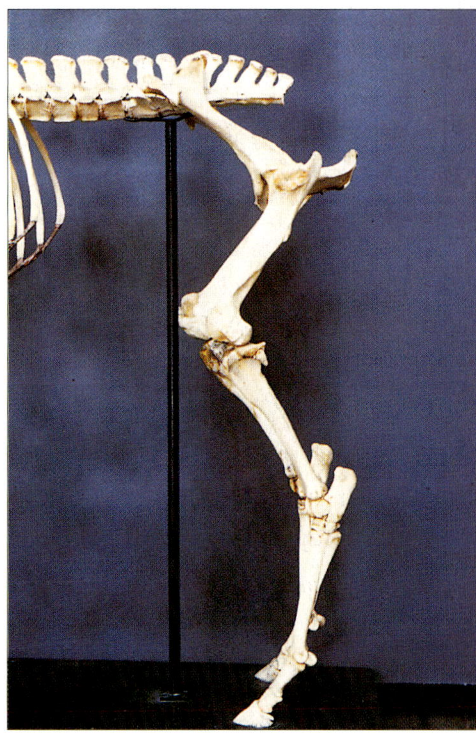

Fig. 138 *The hind leg skeleton*

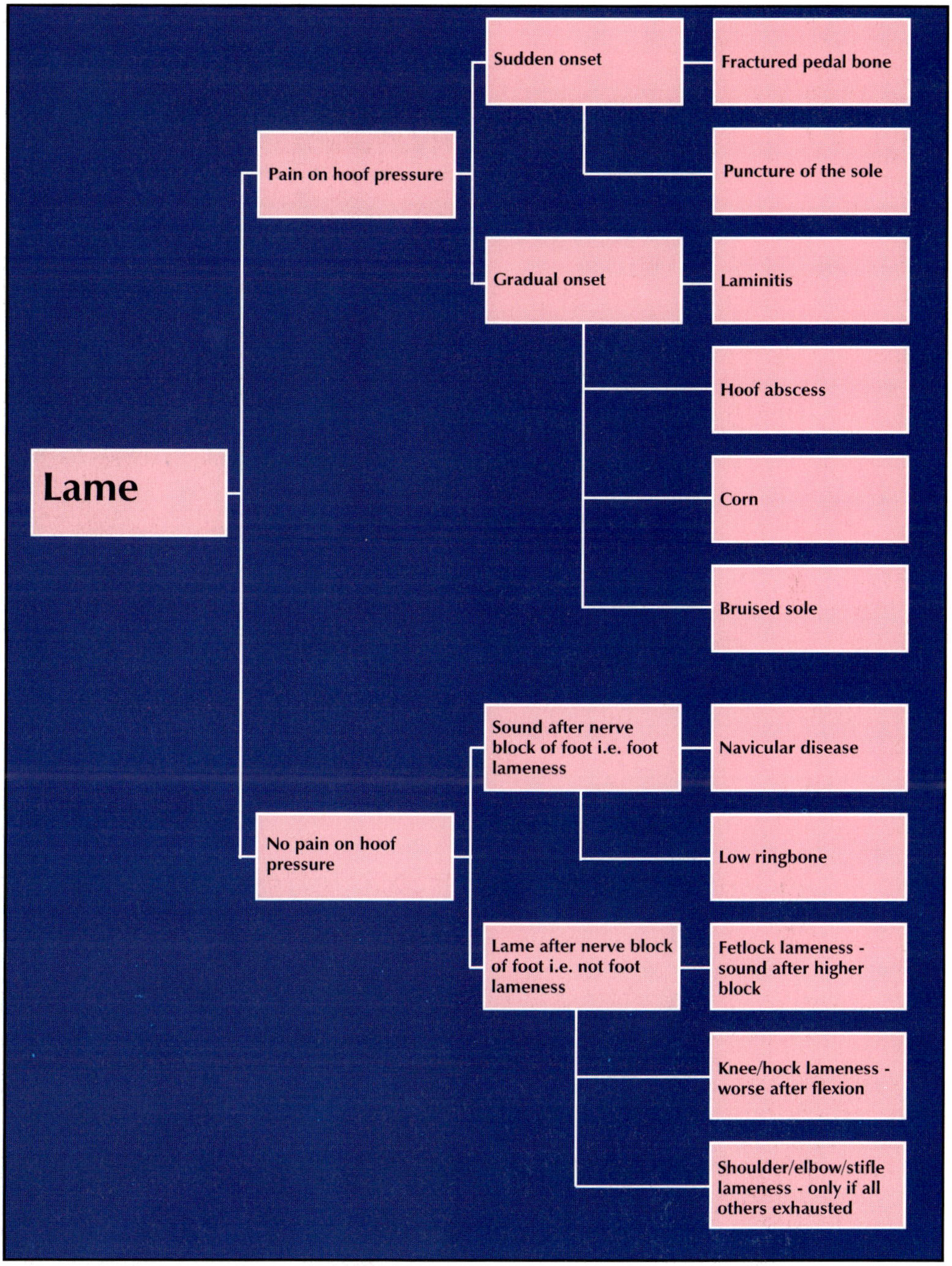

Fig. 139 *The diagnosis of lameness*

design, leaving the muscles of the shoulder exposed to great stress during movement of any kind. It is not surprising that any injury to the shoulder tends to heal slowly. On the other hand it is often the case that injuries to the relatively weak muscles are more common than actual problems with the shoulder joint itself, in much the same way as the safety cut-out on an electrical circuit prevents damage to the appliance itself.

The muscles of the foreleg are all grouped together at the top of the leg, above the knee. They are relatively short and thick, but very powerful. Where necessary, tendons transfer their movement to the bones lower down the leg. The knee joint itself (which is the equivalent of our wrist) consists of many bones, not all of which are involved in movement, but which act as a shock absorber, spreading the stress imparted by the percussive forces of movement over a large number of small bones rather than one large one. This reduces the stress per unit of surface area.

Below the knee there are the three metacarpal bones. During evolution, two of these shrank and now form the splint bones on either side of the cannon bone, which is connected to a single toe, or digit. Behind the fetlock joint are two small pyramid-shaped bones, the sesamoids. They change the direction of the pull of the tendons which attach to them, rather than playing a part in movement of the fetlock joint. A major supply route consisting of an artery, a vein and a nerve runs down the back of the cannon bone, over the fetlock joint and down the pastern. These lie alongside each other, sending off small branches to supply the areas they pass through until they reach the foot.

The foot

Everyone involved with horses knows the expression 'no foot, no horse'. As the foot bears all the weight and provides the movement and contact with the ground, any problem, however small, tends to be reflected in the horse's movement *(Fig. 139)*. The outer part of the foot is the hoof. There is a tendency to consider this as a single protective 'thimble' over the end of the leg, but it does in fact have two distinct parts. The wall of the hoof is separate from the sole although they are firmly stuck together around the white line. The difference is that the horn of the wall grows down from the coronet in tubules. As it grows at a rate of 1.5cm (0.6in) every four to six weeks, the surface of the horn which is worn away by contact with the ground is several months old. The horn over the sole of the foot is laid down over the whole surface. It is only about 2cm (0.8in) thick, so there is a rapid turnover of horn. The practical implication of all this is that a defect of the horn over the sole is replaced relatively quickly, but any damage to the wall of the hoof takes a long time to grow out.

Inside the hoof lies the pedal bone, the last of three bones down the pastern *(Fig. 140)*. The technical problem facing the horse is how to join the keratin protein of the hoof to the bone in such a way that the junction will withstand the terrif-

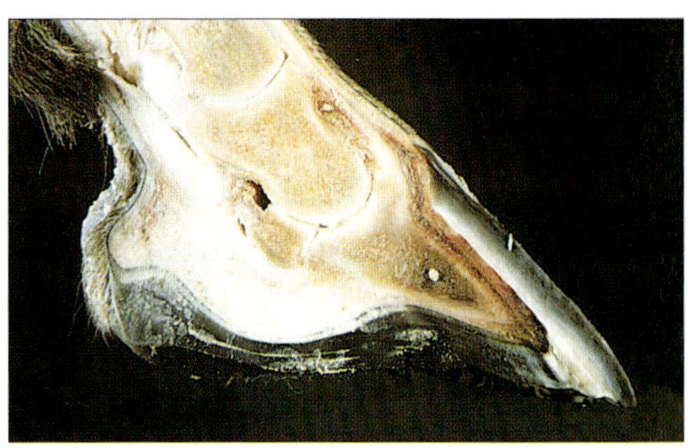

Fig. 140 *An inside view of the horse's foot*
Note particularly the alignment between the central pedal bone and the front hoof wall.

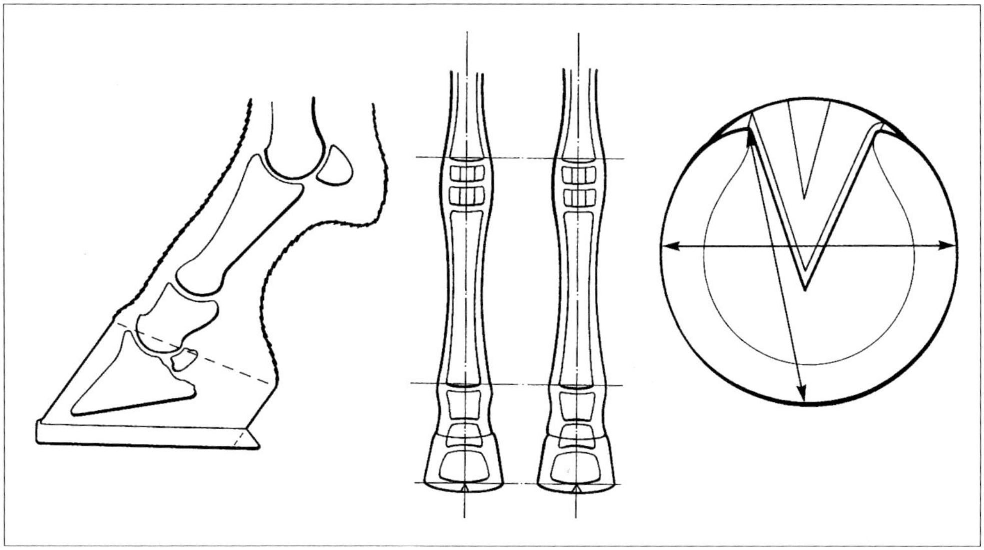

Fig. 141 The measurements which confirm a balanced foot.

ic forces generated when, for example, a horse lands after a jump. The solution is to once again increase the surface area available to absorb the force. The boundary between bone and horn is folded into thousands of interdigitating folds called laminae. The system is so effective that it is even possible to have a layer of tiny blood vessels and nerves between the horn and the bone without the pressure in any one place being so great that it squeezes the blood vessels too much. This plexus of blood vessels is referred to as the sensitive laminae.

The weak spot of the foot is the heel. Here the horn is soft and pliable, and so provides less protection than the rigid wall elsewhere. Ideally this should not matter too much because the lower leg is designed so that the horse's weight, the force of which travels down the centre of the first and second phalanx bones of the pastern, is borne by the centre of the foot. An imaginary force line drawn up the front wall of the hoof continues up the front of the pastern, parallel to another line down the centre of the pastern. This is referred to as a parallel hoof/pastern axis, where the horse's weight is borne forward of the unsupported heel *(Fig. 141)*. Unfortunately, since man assumed responsibility for the shape of the horse's foot by trimming and shoeing it, there has been a tendency to ignore the hoof/pastern axis. Failure to trim enough off the bottom of the hoof at the toe to compensate for natural wear results in a hoof which has a long toe, and a broken (or converging) hoof/pastern axis. The result of this is that the weight is pushed backwards onto the heels. 'Dumping' of the toe, or removing part of the wall around the toe so that there is a vertical section before the natural angle of the hoof does nothing to correct a broken hoof/pastern axis; as far as the forces in the foot are concerned, the toe is still too long and so the weight is still thrown backwards. When looking at the sole of the foot, a line drawn from the angle of the heel to the centre of the toe should be the same length as a line across the widest part of the hoof. If it is, then the hoof is said to to be properly balanced. Failure to balance the foot and maintain a correct hoof/pastern axis is responsible for much of the lameness seen in the leg below the knee.

In addition to the small bones behind the fetlock joint there are other bones

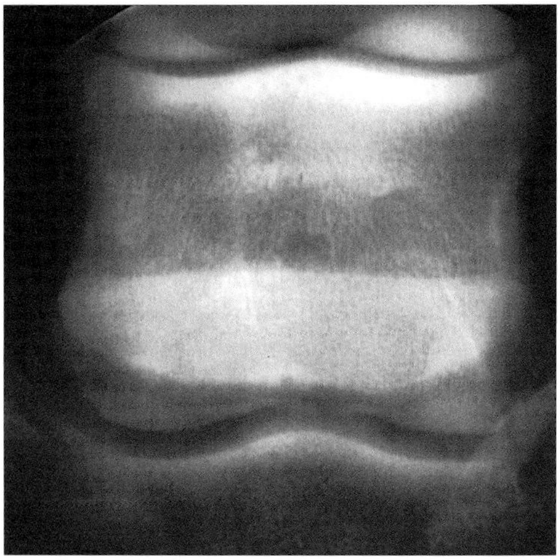

Fig. 142 X-ray of a normal foot showing the navicular bone.

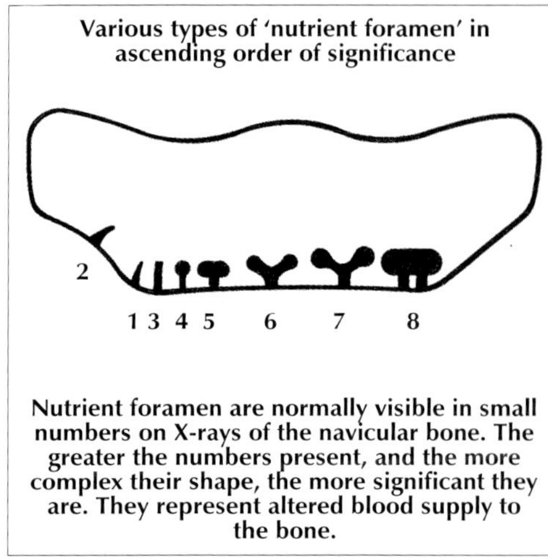

Fig. 143 Diagram showing some of the abnormalities seen on X-rays of the navicular bone in cases of navicular diseases.

which also come into the sesamoid category. There is a sesamoid bone behind the knee joint, for example, and the navicular bone in the foot is also a sesamoid bone. The navicular bone fits neatly into the angle between the back of the pedal bone and the bottom of the second phalanx. It is held in place by two collateral ligaments, each of which runs from the end of the navicular bone to the second phalanx. At the same time the deep flexor tendon, which is responsible for moving the pedal bone backwards, runs over the rear surface of the navicular bone, helping to keep it in place by the quite considerable tension under which that tendon is placed even when the horse is standing still.

Because of the navicular bone's association with lameness, it is important to be aware of the surrounding anatomical features which are also often implicated. The navicular bone receives its blood supply via its bottom edge, the vessels entering the bone through channels called nutrient foramina. These may be visible on X-ray *(Fig. 142)*. Anything which disturbs the blood flow in this heel region may cause the body to increase the size, number or pattern of the nutrient foramina, a fact which we may be able to pick up on X-ray and use to help confirm the site of lameness *(Fig. 143)*.

The blood supply to the foot looks relatively straightforward. An artery runs down either side of the leg as far as the coronet, and a vein running alongside it returns the blood to the general circulation. The main nerve supply also runs alongside these blood vessels. There are two almost separate circulatory systems in the foot, however. One system supplies the coronet and one the pedal bone. We now know that in certain conditions of the foot, the majority of the blood is 'shunted' away from the pedal bone. It goes around the coronet and back up the leg. This causes major problems to the deeper tissues of the foot, which no longer receive as much oxygen as they should do. Much of the pain connected with conditions such as navicular disease, for instance, arises from the anoxia, or oxygen shortage, of the foot following such shunting of blood.

The blood supply to the deeper foot is delivered by a lace-like network of tiny blood vessels which separate the bony laminae of the hoof and the pedal bone. This network is called the sensitive laminae. There is very little blood supply across the 'sole' of the pedal bone, because every time the horse bears weight on the foot these vessels would be squashed. In old books reference is made to the frog cushion acting as a pump to help circulation by squeezing blood out of a plexus of blood vessels beneath the frog every time the foot is put to the ground. We now know that this does not happen because there is very little blood supply underneath the frog. This does not mean a healthy frog does not perform an important role in the foot. It supports the pedal bone, stopping it from squashing the blood vessels over the rest of the sole, and helping to push the bony laminae snugly into the horny laminae.

The hind legs of the horse transfer their propulsive forces to the body via a bony platform called the pelvis. The top bone of the leg, the femur, articulates with the pelvis via a ball and socket joint, the hip joint. It is perhaps worth pointing out that it is not possible to see the horse's hip or to feel it move as a general rule. Both of the bony prominences which we can see on either side of the horse's hind quarters are parts of the pelvis, not the hip. The prominence just in front of the tail is the tuber coxae, and the one further forward is the tuber ischii. The pelvis acts as a platform which literally pushes the spinal column, and the rest of the body, along. There is no true joint between the sacrum of the spine and the pelvis, rather there is a 'groove' in which the spine is held by a very short but very thick ligament called the sacro-iliac ligament.

The femur ends at the stifle joint, which is the equivalent of our knee joint. The horse has a patella, or knee cap, which moves over the end of the femur and the top of tibia. It plays a vital role not performed by the human patella – it is part of the stay apparatus which locks the leg rigid when the horse is standing still. This enables the horse to sleep standing up, an obvious advantage in the wild where it needs to be able to flee from danger at a second's warning. The patella extends medially into a kind of hook. When the horse wants to stand it pulls the patella up via a single tendon from the muscles of the upper leg. Three ligaments (one from each side of the patella and one from the middle) prevent the patella moving too far up because they are attached to the tibia, but they allow sufficient movement for that medial part of the cartilage to be hooked over a bony peg at the bottom of the femur. This effectively fixes the femur and tibia into a set position. The ligaments and tendons of the rest of the horse's leg are so arranged that movement of one joint automatically moves all the other joints. If you flex the stifle joint and look down the leg, you will find that the fetlock joint has also flexed. If you fix the stifle joint, then you fix the other joints. When the horse wants to move, the patella is pulled up and off its peg so that it can move freely again.

The next joint down the leg is the hock joint. Like the 'knee' of the horse this is made up of a number of smaller bones in order to absorb percussion. In fact all the movement at the hock occurs at one joint, between the end of the tibia and the first of three rows of tarsal bones. The rest of the 'joints' between adjacent bones are for shock absorbtion rather than movement. The point of the hock is part of the *os calcis* bone. It acts as a fulcrum to change the direction of pull of the powerful flexor muscles (which attach to it via the achilles tendon) and is the equivalent of our heel. The rest of the hind leg below the hock is basically the same as the front leg below the knee.

Disease prevention

The single most important step in the prevention of lameness and locomotor problems of any sort is to ensure that the horse has properly balanced feet. Some native ponies living wild on the hills achieve this naturally, but most domesticated horses require the regular attention of a qualified farrier. A horse's feet should be trimmed at least every six to eight weeks. If the horse is also shod, the shoes need to be removed for this purpose, no matter how little wear there might be on the shoes themselves. The frequency of shoeing must be dictated by the foot, not by the shoe.

In many parts of the world there is a shortage of farriers, and in all parts of the world there is a shortage of good farriers. In the UK there has traditionally been a tendency for farriers to leave the toe too long. Many horses can survive this, but in others it predisposes to navicular disease, laminitis, joint problems and tendon problems. In the ideal situation, as mentioned above, a horse should have a parallel hoof/pastern axis (i.e. a line drawn up the toe wall of the hoof is parallel to an imaginary line down the centre of the pastern bones) and be balanced so that a line drawn from the heel/frog angle to the centre of the toe is equal in length to a line across the widest part of the foot. If your farrier is unable or unwilling to spend enough time and effort on your horse to produce this, then you should consider finding another one who will. Of course the corollary to this is that horse owners must be prepared to pay farriers enough to justify the time and skill needed to do the job properly. Even when a foot has been properly prepared at the time of shoeing, it will only remain so for 10 to 14 days. After that, hoof growth will begin to unbalance the foot. By 30 to 40 days after trimming the foot will often be unacceptably long.

Each horse is an individual. It follows that we cannot expect half a dozen fixed sizes of manufactured horseshoes to fit every horse properly. Cold shoeing is at best a compromise, and hot shoeing, whether at a fixed or a mobile forge, is required to make the shoe fit the foot. The only exception to making the shoe fit the horse is when the foot already has an abnormality, for example, contracted heels which need to be shod wide in order to encourage the hoof to spread.

The horse's foot is designed to bear the weight on the level bearing surface of the hoof wall. Any studs, which mean an uneven bearing surface, or pads, which spread the weight over the sole as well as the wall, produce abnormal stresses and should be avoided as much as possible. Nature has spent thousands of years perfecting the horse's foot. It is not the shape it is by sheer chance. Nor are we of such superior intellect that we necessarily know better.

Although hoof oils may improve the appearance of the horse's feet, they have little if any effect on the horn itself. They do not penetrate significantly into the hoof wall. In recent times there have been a number of products introduced which are said to improve horn quality. The amino acid D-L Methionine, the vitamin Biotin, and sulphur are all vital for the chemical bridges which hold the horn tubules together. Using one or all of these as supplements may help to improve horn quality, bearing in mind that it takes at least six months to replace the hoof wall.

There is increasing evidence that horses can become 'acclimatised' to quite major physical changes in the locomotor system as long as the demands made on them remain constant. Marked variations in the amount of exercise a horse is given, including periods of complete rest, can result in physical changes giving rise to symptoms. This is why so many horses develop lameness shortly after a change of ownership. Always increase and decrease exercise gradually. It is probably better to give a horse 14 days in a field at one time than to give it one day's complete stable rest per week for 14 weeks.

Azoturia (exertional rhabdomyelitis)

Symptoms In acute cases, the muscles along the back and over the hind quarters become increasingly stiff and painful with exercise. The horse may become 'setfast', unable to move. Because of the pain, symptoms such as sweating, increased respiratory rate, and a raised temperature may be seen. The horse may pass dark-coloured urine, with difficulty. Levels of muscle enzymes in the blood are increased. In sub-acute cases there may be few symptoms other than reduced performance, perhaps with an increased tendency to sweat during exercise.

Cause The localised accumulation of lactic acid in the muscles causes muscle damage. *(Fig. 144).* This may be due to excessive availability of glycogen stored in these muscles from overfeeding. When glycogen is used as a fuel in such circumstances anaerobic metabolism forms lactic acid. There are other considerations involving the effect of of sodium, calcium and chloride levels in the bloodstream upon the sensitivity of muscle cells to damage by lactic acid. Urinary symptoms stem from blockage of the filtering system in the kidneys with the products of muscle breakdown.

Treatment Stop all physical activity as soon as possible to avoid further damage. Exercise should not be restarted until the levels of the muscle enzymes creatinophosphokinase (CPK) and aspartate transferase (AST) circulating in the blood have returned to normal. Reduce feeding until stores of glycogen are used up. Corticosteroids help reduce the inflammation, as does naproxen. Diuretics or intravenous fluids help to wash out the kidneys. Vitamin E is said by some to be useful. Sodium, calcium and chloride supplementation in the diet may help to prevent further attacks. The precise need for supplementation in an individual horse over and above the food levels normally considered adequate can be measured by a creatine clearance test. This measures the proportion of electrolytes being excreted in the urine compared with blood levels. A horse will remain susceptible to azoturia until the creatine clearance becomes normal, no matter how well the horse looks externally.

Prognosis Good as long as the predisposing circumstances are not repeated – chiefly over-feeding relative to the amount of exercise.

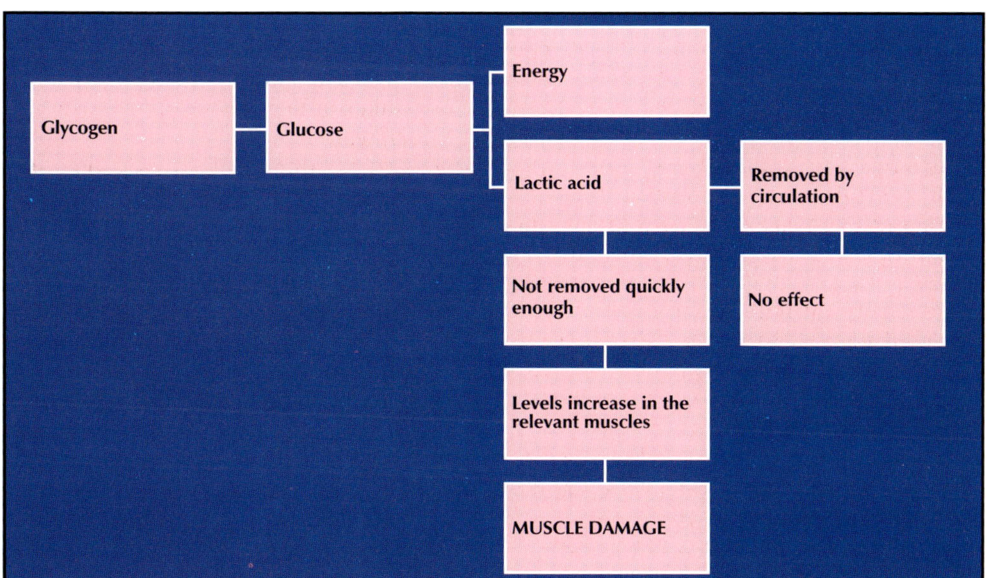

Fig. 144 *Muscle damage in azoturia*

Back problems

Symptoms The horse has reduced performance. It may have an altered action. There may be wasting of the muscles *(Fig. 145)*. Localised spasms of the *longissimus dorsi* muscle along the spine result in pain when the affected spot is pressed.

Cause Often there is muscle damage alone. In other cases the vertebrae of the spine are also involved. The most common such problem is when adjacent dorsal spines come to rub against each other. Note that the vertebrae are not displaced or out of alignment.

Treatment Manipulation, laser, ultrasonic and faradic treatments have all been used to relax the muscle spasm. Rest alone may allow resolution of any bony condition. Surgery, e.g. removal of rubbing dorsal spines, may be needed.

Prognosis Fair, but often no attempt is made to look for the underlying cause of such problems, e.g. a lameness elsewhere which is causing the horse to transfer its weight abnormally via the spine.

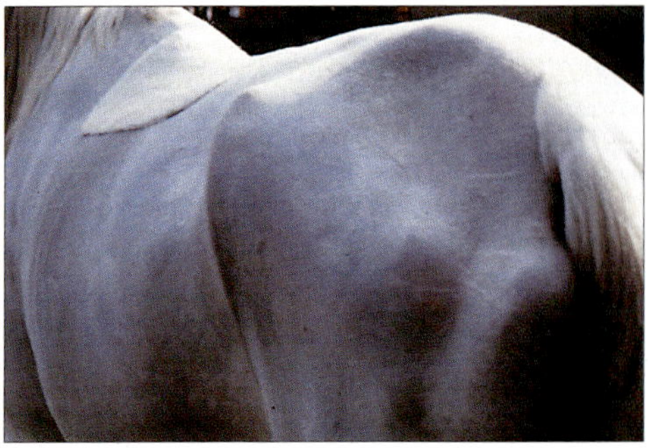

Fig. 145 Marked muscle wasting over the hind quarters in a horse with a back problem.

Bog spavin

Symptoms A distinct fluid-filled swelling appears on one or both sides of the hock joint. It is not painful and does not cause lameness. Pressure on one of the swellings can be felt to increase pressure in the swelling on the other side of the joint. It is not associated with true spavin (see page 167), despite its name.

Cause Increase in fluid produced by the joint capsule, but the capsule can only expand in these specific areas because elsewhere it is constricted by ligaments, for example. It is usually a response to an injury.

Treatment Complete rest and pressure bandaging are recommended. Laser therapy may help resolve the swelling. Cortisone injections may be effective but carry great risk for the joint as a whole.

Prognosis Good in acute cases but poor once the condition becomes established.

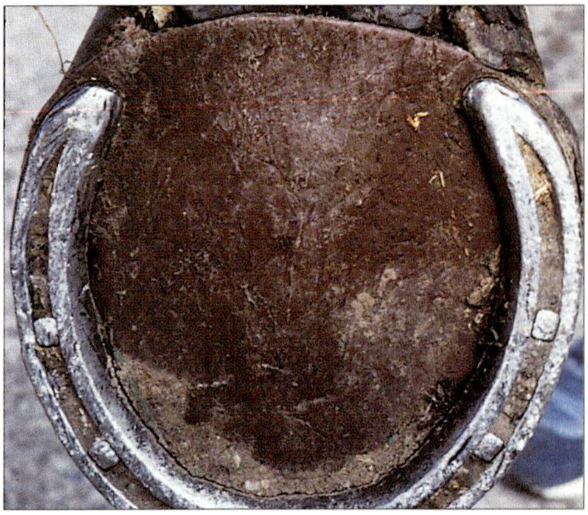

Fig. 146 A leather pad fitted underneath the shoe to protect the sole of the foot.

Bruised sole

Symptoms The horse is moderately lame with no visible cause. Careful examination of the sole with the shoe removed may reveal a reddish discoloration around the white line.

Cause A poorly-fitting shoe can bruise the sole. Treading on a hard object which fails to puncture the sole can cause bruising, especially in horses with thin soles or poor quality horn.

Treatment Rest is essential. The temporary fitting of a soft pad over the sole may ease the discomfort by preventing further pressure *(Fig. 146)*. Pain-killing drugs have little effect, but corticosteroids may help to reduce the bruising slightly.

Prognosis Good.

Bursitis

Symptoms Distinct soft painless swellings over joints, usually over the front surface of a joint such as the fetlock.

Cause A bursa is a hollow 'cushion' which usually contains very little fluid. Considerably more fluid is produced in an attempt to cushion a joint or tendon and protect it from trauma.

Treatment Pressure bandaging and cold applications can cause a rapid shrinking of the swollen bursa. The fluid may be drained out and corticosteroid injected into the bursa. It is possible in some cases to remove the bursa surgically.

Prognosis Guarded. The swelling often remains, even though it is not interfering with movement, and does not cause lameness unless acutely inflamed.

Capped hock

Symptoms A non-painful fluid-filled swelling just over the point of the hock *(Fig. 147)*. The horse is not lame unless the swelling is very large.

Cause This is a specific form of bursitis caused by trauma, for example during travelling, or if there is insufficient bedding in the stable.

Treatment Cold applications and a pressure bandage are applied. The fluid can be drained out of the bursa and replaced by a small amount of long-acting corticosteroid.

Prognosis May become chronic and unresponsive if cause persists.

Check ligament desmitis

Symptoms Lameness associated with swelling of the upper third of the flexor tendons. Ultrasound scan may confirm the diagnosis.

Cause A sprain of the check ligament fibres or their attachment to the flexor tendon.

Treatment Cold and rest may result in a rapid improvement, although recurrence is common when the horse returns to work. Otherwise as for sprains of tendons (see page 168).

Prognosis Good at first occurrence, but, once established, guarded, especially for a return to jumping.

Club foot

Symptoms One or more feet are very upright in the angle of the hoof wall to the ground *(Fig. 148)*.

Cause The basic cause is a contraction of the deep digital flexor tendon. This may be an inherited problem. It may be associated with nutritional deficiencies in young horses. It may be due to injury.

Treatment The main treatment is correction of any nutritional problems. Foot trimming may help.

Prognosis Poor.

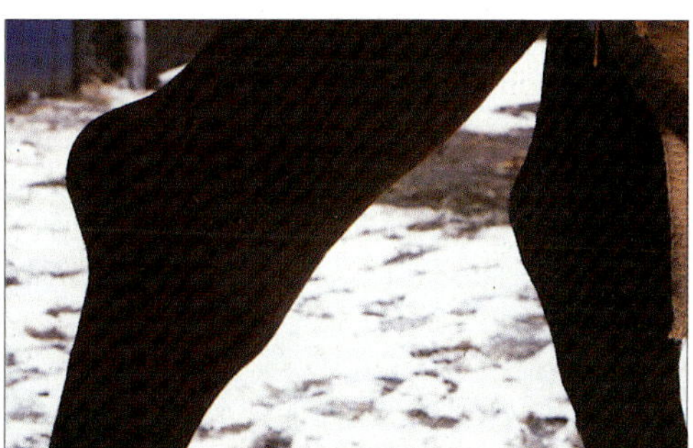

Fig. 147 *A capped hock*

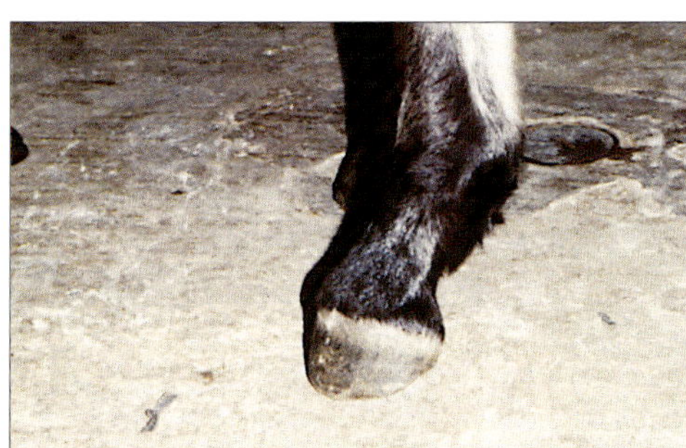

Fig. 148 *Club foot*
The foot is upright and contracted.

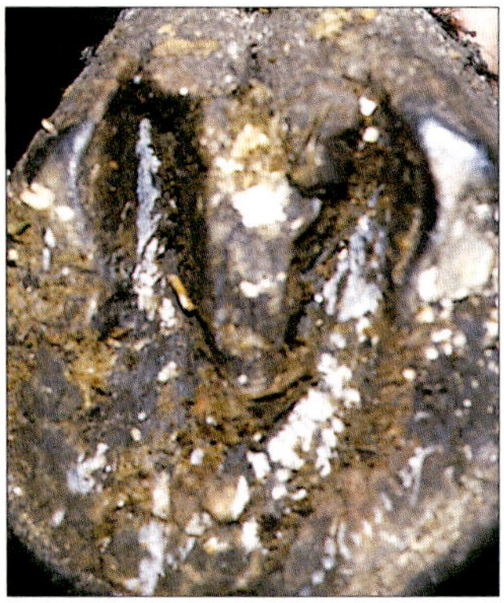

Fig. 149 *Corns*
The hoof has obviously been neglected.

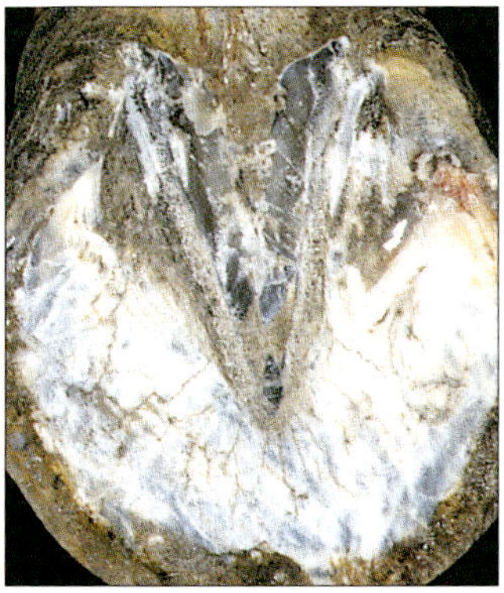

Fig. 150 *A corn*
The discolored area is visible just to the right of the frog.

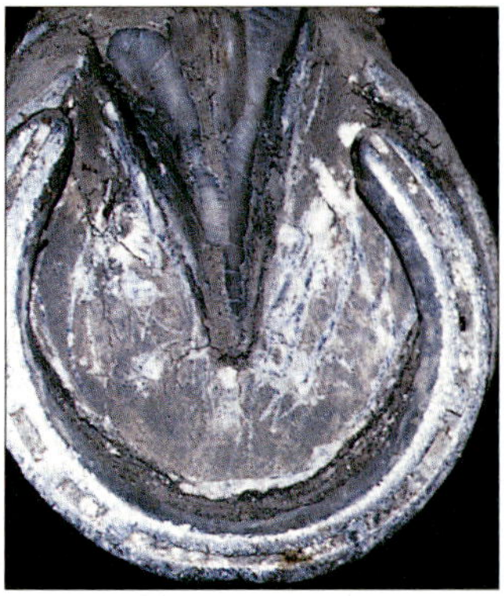

Fig. 151 *Poorly fitting shoe pressing on the seat of a corn*

Corn

Symptoms The horse is chronically lame. Pressure over the seat of the corn is painful. When the shoe is removed and the horn pared, red bruising of the horn can be seen. If the corn is infected, black pus can be seen *(Figs. 149 & 150)*. The inside of the front feet are most commonly affected.

Cause Pressure from a badly-fitting shoe on the sole *(Fig. 151)*.

Treatment The bruised horn is cut away. Poulticing for one or two days is followed by the fitting of a shoe with cut away heels on the ground surface over the seat of the corn. The cavity may be plugged with Stockholm tar and cotton wool to prevent infection or the lodging of gravel.

Prognosis Good.

Curb

Symptoms A ridge-like swelling appears on the back of a hind leg just below the hock *(Fig. 152)*. Initial lameness may be increased by the spavin test (see page 167). In time the condition becomes painless.

Cause When it affects both legs or occurs in young horses, the underlying cause is often faulty conformation. The swelling is due to a thickening of the plantar ligament between adjacent bones in the hock. Over-extension of the hock joint when trying to pull up suddenly from the gallop may cause an acute reaction in older horses.

Treatment If treatment is necessary in an acute case, a combination of DMSO and cortisone can be applied to the skin over the curb. The heels of the shoe should be raised slightly.

Prognosis Fair as it often causes no lameness, especially in non-jumping animals.

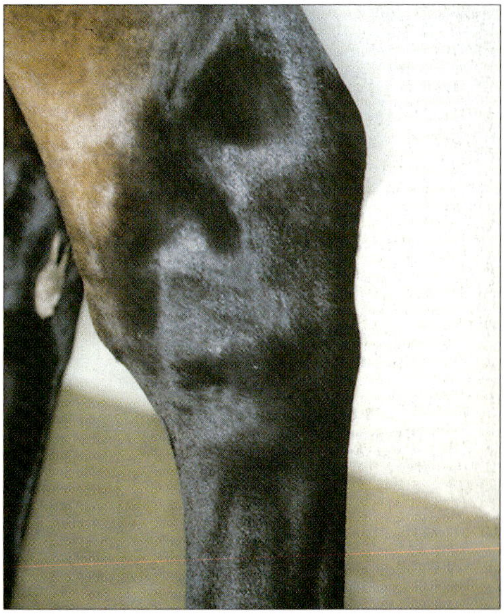

Fig. 152 *A curb*

Degenerative joint disease
Symptoms This term can apply to any joint of the body, although the fetlock, knee and hock joints are most commonly affected. The joint capsule is swollen and puffy. It may initially be warm to the touch, but cools as time passes. The horse has varying degrees of lameness, often exacerbated by forced flexion of the joint. X-rays may reveal bony changes to the joint surfaces *(Fig. 153)*.

Cause Wear and tear. Inflammation of the membrane lining the joint capsules results in the production of an ineffective joint fluid and 'decay' of the joint surfaces it normally keeps healthy.

Treatment Cold and pressure bandaging is used during the initial inflammation. Anti-inflammatory drugs and therapy are useful. Replacement of the reduced quality joint fluid with synthetic fluid of normal viscosity can bring about a speedy recovery. Such joints may remain relatively pain-free with a constant level of exercise but become painful when exercise is started again after a period of rest, or with increased exercise for some other reason, for example, a new owner.

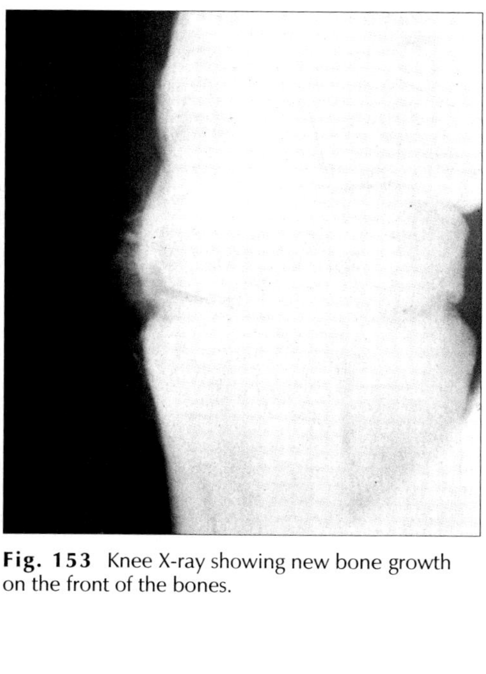

Fig. 153 Knee X-ray showing new bone growth on the front of the bones.

A constant level of exercise should therefore be maintained. Polyamino glycans injected into the joint or intramuscularly may protect the joint cartilage from damage and allow healing.

Prognosis Fair unless permanent bony changes have occurred.

Fistulous withers
Symptoms Heat and swelling over the withers is followed by a discharge of pus.

Cause Badly-fitting tack causes bruising, and infection gains entry into the affected tissue. Thankfully, less common than in years gone by.

Treatment Surgery may be necessary to remove necrotic (dead) tissue. The wound is washed with sloughing agents to promote proper healing. Antibiotic therapy needs to be prolonged.

Prognosis Fair.

Fractures
Symptoms A sudden onset of lameness. Depending on the bone involved, there may be a marked abnormality of limb shape and a complete inability to bear weight.

Cause Trauma.

Treatment For repair to take place, all bone fragments have to be completely immobilised – either by a rigid cast of some sort or by using metal screws and plates to repair the fracture surgically.

Prognosis The prognosis for all fractures above the knee or hock is grave except in very young foals. The prognosis for fractures of the knee and hock is fair with surgery. The prognosis for fractures below the knee and hock is fair with surgery unless it is a comminuted fracture (i.e. with several fragments), when it is poor. The prognosis for compound, or open fractures, i.e. where a bone fragment has penetrated the skin through to the outside and possibly become contaminated, is always grave.

Fracture of the navicular bone

Symptoms Usually a sudden increase of the symptoms of navicular disease (see page 161). Can be due to trauma. The fracture is visible on X-ray.

Cause Weakening of the bone may be a result of pre-existing navicular disease, especially if the problem has been masked by the use of phenylbutazone.

Treatment Surgery has been attempted by screwing together the fragments.

Prognosis Poor.

Fracture of the splint bone

Symptoms Acute lameness is accompanied by marked pain over the splint bone. The area is warm and swollen at first, but this may resolve leaving just a hard swelling over the bone. The lameness may improve with rest, only to reappear when the horse returns to strenuous exercise.

Cause Stress fractures can occur. They usually only affect part of the thickness of the bone. Fractures right through the bone are usually the result of a blow, such as a kick.

Treatment Rest, with or without pulsed electromagnetic therapy, may allow the bone to heal. If the fracture is completely through the bone, it is often advisable to remove the fragment surgically and then to anchor the body of the splint bone to the cannon bone with a screw.

Prognosis Good.

Hyperflexion of the limbs

Symptoms The angle of the fetlock is much straightened in one or more legs *(Fig. 154)*. The heel of the foot may be raised from the ground. Eventually the fetlock passes over the vertical with regard to the foot. Most commonly seen in young growing horses.

Cause Poor trimming of the feet, poor conformation and inadequate exercise may predispose to the condition. Both overfeeding and imbalanced feeding at a time of rapid bone growth are often involved.

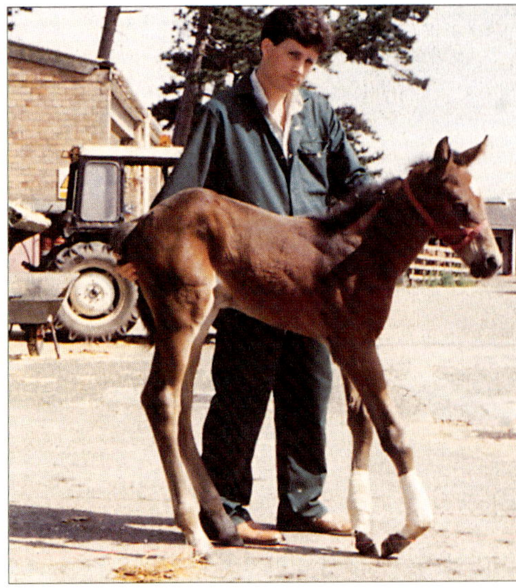

Fig. 154 *Hyperflexion of the limbs*
The fetlocks are straightened or knuckled over.

Treatment A drastic reduction should be made in the food consumed (including grazing). Trimming of the foot involves lowering of the heels relative to the toes. A special shoe with a toe extension helps to keep the heels down on the ground. Surgical correction may be necessary, cutting the check ligament which normally restricts the flexor tendons.

Prognosis Guarded.

Infected joint wounds

Symptoms The joint is hot and swollen. Sudden onset of marked lameness. Puncture wound may or may not be visible. The horse may have a raised temperature. Chronic damage to cartilage and bone visible on X-ray.

Cause Wound allowing infection access to the joint capsule.

Treatment In acute stage profuse flushing of the joint with saline, possibly under general anaesthetic. Prolonged antibiotic therapy.

Prognosis Guarded. Condition may appear to respond but then recur.

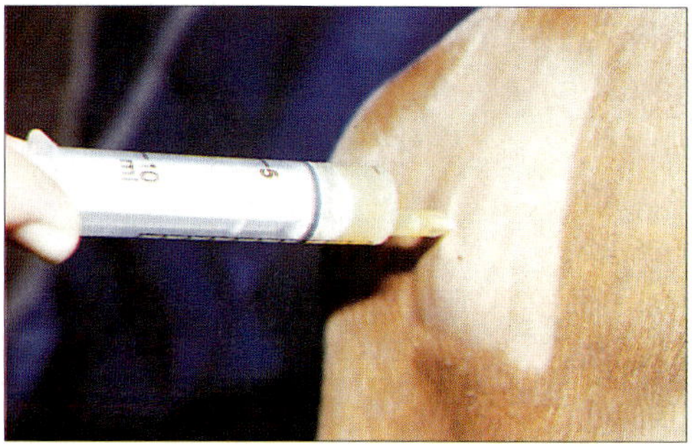

Fig. 155 *Joint ill*
Withdrawing pus from the affected joint.

Joint ill

Symptoms Usually more than one joint is affected, in foals of two to three months and under. The joint is swollen, hot and very painful *(Fig. 155)*. The foal has a high temperature.

Cause Bacteria gain entry to the joint capsule from the bloodstream. In very young foals they often enter the body via the navel. Bacteria may be cultured from the joint.

Treatment Prompt treatment with antibiotics is essential, based as soon as possible on sensitivity tests on the bacteria. Irrigation of the affected joints may be beneficial.

Prognosis The larger the number of joints affected, the poorer the prognosis.

Laminitis

Symptoms Heat in the hoof of one or more feet, lameness and distortion of the hoof involving rotation of the pedal bone. May have dietary origin.

For full details see page 76.

Myositis

Symptoms The affected muscle is swollen, painful and may feel warm.

Cause Trauma, either tearing by an uncoordinated movement or bruising from a fall.

Treatment Cold and rest initially. Physiotherapy may be beneficial.

Prognosis Good as long as the horse is not put back into work until the inflammation has subsided. Muscle enzyme levels may help to determine when this point has been reached.

Nail bind

Symptoms Pain and lameness on shoeing.

Cause Pressure on the sensitive laminae of the foot from a poorly placed nail.

Treatment The nail must be removed. Poulticing and antibiotic therapy may be necessary if there is any infection.

Prognosis Good.

Navicular disease

Symptoms Intermittent lameness progresses to continuous lameness of one or both front feet. The horse may stumble occasionally. Initially the lameness may wear off with exercise but is more marked following 30 minutes rest after exercise. Flexion of the foot may increase the lameness. Occasionally, navicular disease may lead to contraction of the heels so that the foot looks smaller than its opposite foot. X-ray examination shows changes in the navicular bone, although the severity of these changes bears no correlation to the degree of lameness. Changes seen include an increase in nutrient foramina and the presence of abnormally-shaped foramina.

Cause Navicular disease is as much a problem of blood pressure in the foot as of bone changes. Poor shoeing, particularly when it results in a long toe, increases pressure in the heel region, interfering with circulation around the foot. Any change in work, environment or shoeing can trigger the symptom.

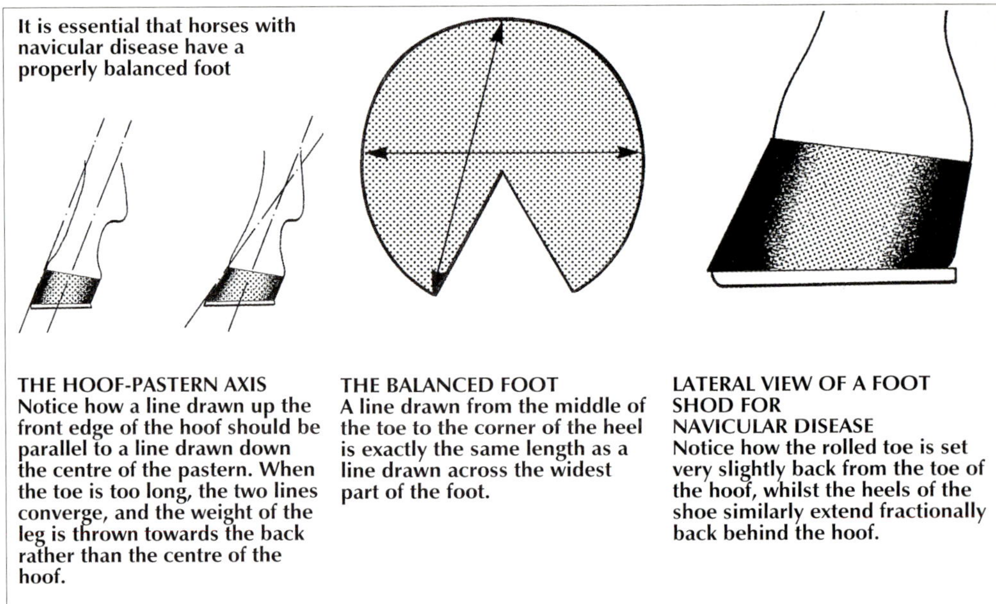

Fig. 156 *Assessing the foot in the prevention of navicular disease*
A properly balanced foot with a parallel hoof/pastern axis and shod as shown is much less likely to develop navicular disease.

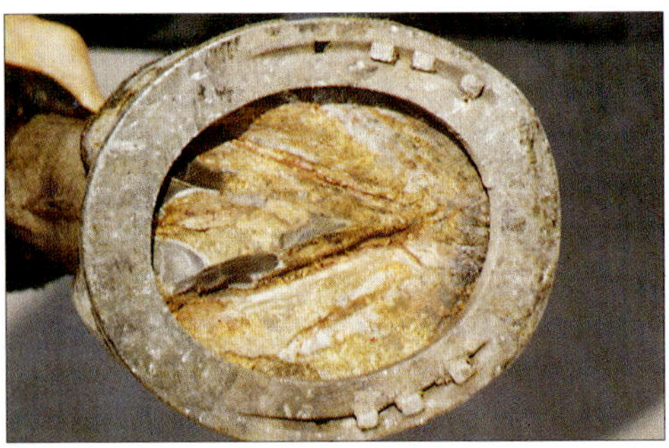

Fig. 157 *An eggbar shoe*

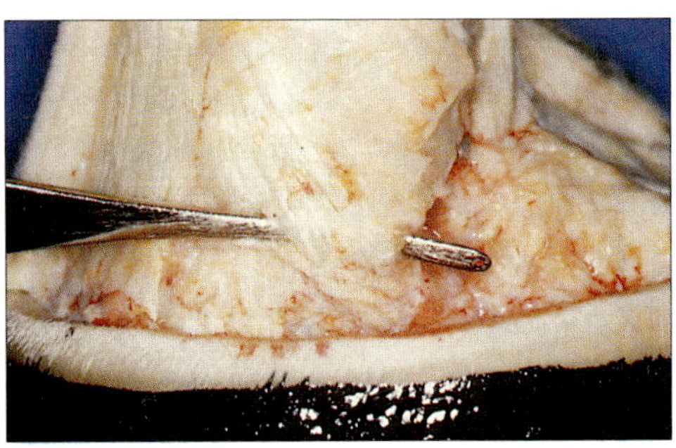

Fig. 158 *The collateral ligament which holds the navicular bone*
This ligament is severed in a desmotomy operation to treat navicular disease.

Treatment Correct shoeing with a rolled toe set back and possibly a bar at the heel is essential. *(Figs. 156 & 157)* Drugs which increase the peripheral blood supply such as warfarin (which is toxic and needs constant monitoring) and isoxsuprine (which is non-toxic) bring relief from lameness. This relief may well be permanent, although the changes in the navicular bone remain. Painkilling drugs such as phenylbutazone have previously been frequently used to mask the symptoms and allow the horse to return to work. Neurectomy (cutting the nerve which supplies the foot) has also been used *(Fig. 158)*. Surgical cutting of the collateral ligaments to the navicular bone (desmotomy) may result in a return to soundness as the bone can then settle into a better position relative to the surrounding structures.

Prognosis With modern treatment 60-70% of horses return to work and require no further treatment other than attention to shoeing.

Osteochondrosis

Symptoms A sudden onset of lameness in a young horse or one only recently starting strenuous work. One or more joints may be affected, with the stifle, hock and fetlocks most commonly involved. The joint capsule may be distended with increased joint fluid. On X-ray a piece of detached bone may be seen floating loose in the joint or there may be a flap-like lesion on a bone surface. It may also be seen arthroscopically.

Cause Interference in the metabolism of the cartilage ossifying into bone during the first six months or so of life. The resultant line of weakness later gives way under stress.

Treatment If a detached bone fragment is present it should be removed surgically. Affected areas of cartilage should be scraped clean surgically, so the resulting cavity can fill with healthy cartilage.

Prognosis Good if surgical treatment is carried out successfully. If not diagnosed, may result in degenerative joint disease (see page 159).

Pedal ostitis

Symptoms This has been called a radiographic disease. The specific changes which show up on X-ray are a rarefaction of areas of the pedal bone, but these are of uncertain significance. The horse may or may not be lame.

Cause Early navicular disease or laminitis are usually the cause of the changes, i.e. diseases which interfere with blood flow in the feet.

Treatment Treatment for the real cause is necessary.

Prognosis Good if this is the only change present.

Poll evil

Symptoms The horse resents bending and movement of its head. There may be a painful swelling on either side of the poll area.

Cause It has been associated with pressure from tight tack. *Onchocerca* (see page 117) has infested the area, giving rise to the development of a fistula or channel through which fluid drains to the skin surface. Brucellosis infection of the atlantal bursa in the poll has occurred.

Treatment If necessary, specific treatment is carried out for any *onchocerca* or brucellosis infections. Anti-inflammatory treatment is important, and the horse must not be worked as this involves 'collection', or bending, of the neck.

Prognosis Fair.

Punctured sole

Symptoms The horse may be acutely lame, hardly willing to put its foot to the ground at all. Heat is often present, and the horse resents pressure to its sole, especially around the affected area. Careful examination of the hoof reveals a black mark which when it is cut away exposes pus. Ascending infection may result in puffiness of the pastern and lower leg.

Cause Penetration of the sole by any sharp object causes infection, especially by anaerobic bacteria.

Treatment The hole must be enlarged to allow adequate drainage. Poulticing is carried out until no more pus is evident. Metronidazole is effective at killing anaerobic bacteria which might otherwise persist. The hole must be plugged or otherwise protected to prevent further infection. Systemic antibiotics may prevent spread or continuation of infection.

Prognosis Good.

Quittor

Symptoms Swelling and pain at the coronet over the lateral cartilage. Pus discharges from a hole which then heals, only for the pus to break out elsewhere. The horse is lame.

Cause An area of infected necrotic tissue in the lateral cartilage, which may be the result of damage to the coronary band or may be due to an infection penetrating up from the sole.

Treatment Surgery should be carried out to remove the necrotic cartilage.

Prognosis Good.

Rickets

Symptoms This is a condition which can affect one or several bones in an immature horse. The ends of the affected bone become painful and swollen over the epiphysis or growth plate. The bone may become deformed. Besides affecting its movement, rickets results in the horse becoming dull. Levels of the enzyme alkaline phosphatase in the blood are increased, but mineral levels may be normal. Bone changes are visible on X-ray.

Cause The abnormal bone has low levels of calcium and phosphorus. This may be due to a deficiency in the diet but it can also be due to reduced absorption by damaged intestines. Lack of Vitamin D exacerbates the problem.

Treatment Correct levels of calcium (6g/100 kg bodyweight) and phosphorus (4g/100 kg bodyweight) must be given. Extra Vitamin D may be necessary in the winter (normally manufactured in the horse's skin by the action of sunlight).

Prognosis Good, unless deformity of the skeleton has taken place.

Ringbone

Symptoms The horse is lame and the lameness may be increased by flexing the foot. A hard bony swelling may be felt at the joint between the first and second phalanxes (high ringbone) or between the second and third phalanxes (low ringbone). On the X-ray, new bone can be seen around the respective joint *(Fig. 159)*. So-called non-articular ringbone involves deposition of new bone around the ligaments well away from a joint.

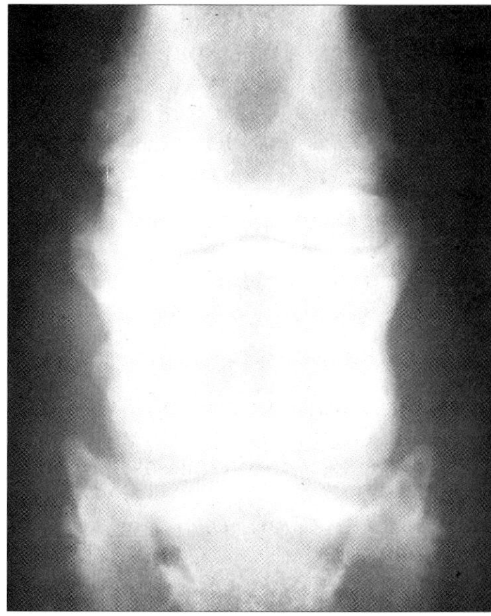

Fig. 159 *X-ray showing ringbone*
Note the fuzzy outline around the joint due to new bone formation.

Cause Ringbone is a disease of wear and tear. Poor hoof care and balancing may be contributory factors.

Treatment There is no cure. Pain-killing drugs such as phenylbutazone may relieve the lameness temporarily. Attention to shoeing is important.

Prognosis Poor for articular ringbone. Non-articular ringbone may become symptomless in time.

Ruptured Achilles tendon

Symptoms The hock of the affected leg is lower to the ground, so that the angle of the hock is always increased, and it cannot be straightened. The horse may not be able to bear any weight on the leg.

Cause Trauma to the tendon. If only the gastrocnemius tendon as it approaches the point of the hock is ruptured, the leg will still be able to bear some weight. If the superficial flexor tendon is also ruptured at the same place, the horse will not be able to use the leg at all.

Treatment The horse needs a cast down the full length of the leg. An attempt may be made to suture the ends of the ruptured tendons together.

Prognosis Poor.

Sacro-iliac strain

Symptoms Reduced performance may become even more obvious as training for suppleness is increased. Lameness is not usually present. Wasting of the gluteal muscle on the affected side causes a visible asymmetry when the horse is examined from behind *(Fig. 160)*. Pressure on the gluteal muscles produces pain.

Cause The sacro-iliac ligament may be sprained during rolling or jumping etc. The gluteal muscles which attach in this area cause pain if they contract and pull on the ligament.

Treatment Complete stable rest is essential initially. Any secondary problems such as muscular spasms must also be dealt with. If treatment is unsuccessful, performance may be regained on permanent analgesic therapy using a very carefully controlled programme of increasing exercise.

Prognosis Poor. The condition tends to recur when training increases in intensity again.

Sandcrack

Symptoms A vertical crack in the wall of the hoof *(Fig.161)*. Usually it starts at the weight-bearing surface and extends up towards the coronet. The horse may or may not be lame.

Cause Drying out of the outer layer of the hoof wall and poor quality horn may trigger the crack. Once it reaches the coronet, damage to the horn-forming cells means that the crack is self-perpetuating. Lameness is caused by movement of the hoof wall on the sensitive laminae.

Treatment The two sides of the crack must be stabilised. Horizontal grooving across the top of the crack will stop it spreading upwards only if the groove is deeper than the sandcrack. Vertical grooves on either side of the sandcrack

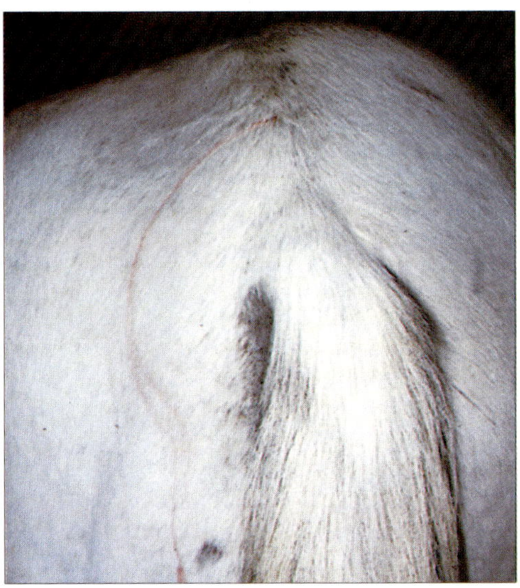

Fig. 160 *Sacro-illiac strain*
Note the marked muscle wastage over the affected side.

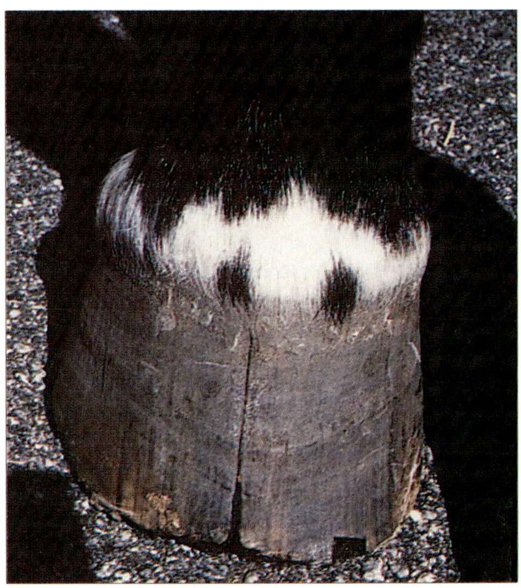

Fig. 161 *A sandcrack*

reduce the torsion forces in the hoof wall. Full stabilisation of the crack may require cleaning away of infected horn and stabilisation with artificial horn material.

Prognosis Good if treatment is active. Will take up to six months for crack to grow out.

Seedy toe

Symptoms Lameness may be intermittent. Examination of the sole reveals dark-coloured crumbling horn around the white line at the toe. This may extend a considerable distance into the foot.

Cause Long toes and poor quality horn predispose to separation of the white line. Dirt and stones can become impacted upwards, forming a wedge.

Treatment All the infected horn must be cut away, no matter how deep. The cavity can then be filled with synthetic horn after cleaning with metronidazole to kill any remaining anaerobic bacteria.

Prognosis Good.

Sesamoiditis

Symptoms The sesamoid bones behind the fetlock may be painful when pressed. The changes in the bones may cause lameness, but often only affect stride length and performance. The condition is often chronic.

Cause There are changes in the structure of the bones (visible on X-ray) as a result of excessive pulling forces from the flexor tendons. Fracture of the bone may occur.

Treatment Rest and cold applications are recommended. Fractures do not heal well, even with surgery.

Prognosis Guarded in chronic cases and poor if a fracture has occurred.

Shoulder sprain

Symptoms Most symptoms attributed to shoulder lameness are due to lameness elsewhere. When the joint is injured, movement is painful. The muscles waste away. The horse is lame, especially when walking in a circle or on a hill.

Cause Trauma, often caused by a bad landing after a jump.

Treatment Routine anti-inflammatory treatments are used. Up to six months' rest may be necessary if the shoulder is to be able to recover completely. Physiotherapy is essential.

Prognosis Good as long as no permanent damage to the joint has occurred.

Side bone

Symptoms The lateral cartilages become ossified and may be felt to have lost their elasticity where they extend above the coronet at the heels. The new bone can be seen on X-rays. Lameness is rare in riding horses *(Fig. 162)*.

Cause With age the lateral cartilages may naturally become ossified, and excessive percussion can speed up this process.

Treatment Correct shoeing is essential if lameness is present. Vertical grooving of

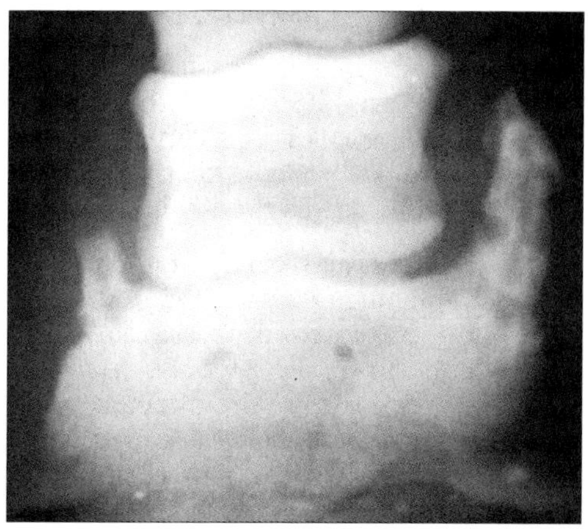

Fig. 162 *Side bone*
Note how the corner of the pedal bone extends upwards due to new bone formation in the lateral cartilage.

the hoof wall over the quarters may relieve the pressure.

Prognosis Good as few symptoms.

Sore shins or bucked shins
Symptoms If both shins are affected the horse may not be lame but merely have a very shortened stride. The front of the cannon bone is warm to the touch. It may be painful. Almost entirely a problem of immature horses.

Cause The inflammation of the bone is due to an inability of the immature bone to withstand the stresses of work.

Treatment Rest removes the stress. Laser or pulsing electro-magnetic therapy may speed healing.

Prognosis Good.

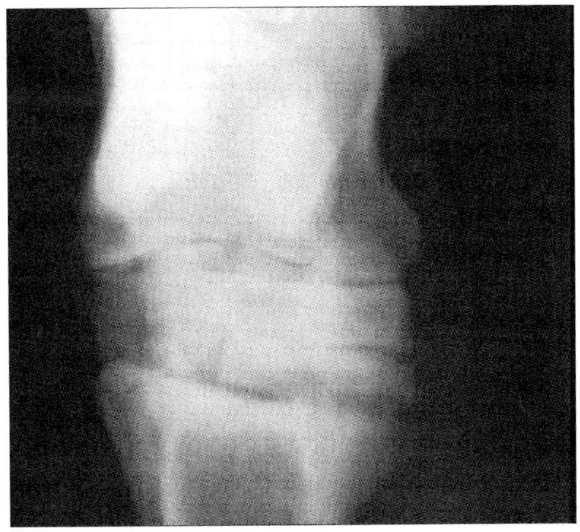

Fig. 163 *Spavin*
New bone is formed around the joints between the layers of small bones in the hock.

Spavin
Symptoms Hind leg lameness with shortening of the stride. The lameness may be more pronounced after standing. It may be markedly increased by holding the leg up with the hock joint flexed for 20 to 30 seconds and then trotting the horse straight away (the 'spavin test'). Only occasionally can a hard bony swelling be seen on the inside of the hock. On X-ray, changes can be seen between the small bones of the hock *(Fig. 163)*.

Cause Wear and tear on the joints between the small bones of the hock is exacerbated by poor conformation and shoeing. Spavin is a chronic osteoarthritis of the joints within the hock.

Treatment Corrective shoeing prevents the leg being angled under the horse thus increasing the uneven pressures in the joint. With continued exercise (perhaps using analgesic drugs) the affected joints may fuse together. Once this happens the horse becomes sound. This fusion may also be achieved surgically. Some relief may be obtained by cutting the cunean tendon as it runs over the medial hock.

Prognosis Guarded.

Splints
Symptoms Initially the horse may be lame without any visible cause. More usually a hard, painful swelling can be felt on the cannon bone/splint bone junction. Splints are commonest on the inside of the leg, on the front legs and in young horses. They can, however, occur in old horses. They can also appear without causing any lameness.

Cause The swelling consists of new bone and fibrous tissue laid down by the surface covering, or periosteum, of the cannon bone. It is considered an attempt to strengthen the bone to withstand the stresses of percussion.

Treatment Rest removes the percussion already mentioned. Cortisone injected locally or applied to the skin with DMSO may reduce the inflammation. Laser therapy or pulsing electromagnetic therapy may speed healing. Very large splints can be removed surgically.

Prognosis Good. Splints rarely cause any trouble once they have settled down, although the swelling remains. Surgical removal may be followed by some regrowth of the splint.

Sprained tendons

Symptoms The tendon and its tendon sheath (almost always the flexor tendons down the back of the cannon) are swollen and enlarged *(Fig. 164)*. The swelling is initially hot and painful, becoming cold in time. Lameness depends on the severity of the condition and the time since it occurred. Ultrasound scanning may show the extent of the damage in the structure of the tendon *(Figs. 165 & 166)*.

Cause Excessive tension on the tendons usually occurs when the horse is tired, perhaps due to a lack of fitness, or makes a sudden uncoordinated movement.

Treatment Rest is essential. Initially, cold and pressure bandages are used to relieve the initial inflammation. Laser therapy is effective in reducing the swelling. Various surgical techniques are said to improve healing (e.g. tendon-splitting and/or carbon fibre implants), and reduce tension in the tendons (e.g. check ligament desmotomy). Firing tendons with a hot iron, widely practised in the past, has now largely been discontinued. Prompt treatment with polysulphated glycosaminoglycan may speed up the repair rate of injured tendon tissue.

Prognosis Depends on the severity of the injury. In severe sprains the prognosis is poor, and complete rupture of the tendon may occur. In this case there is marked sinking of the affected fetlock leg when the horse stands square *(Fig. 167)*.

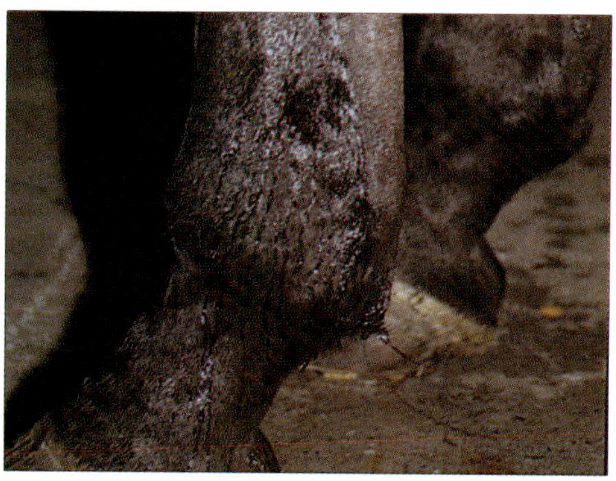

Fig. 164 *A sprained, or bowed, tendon*

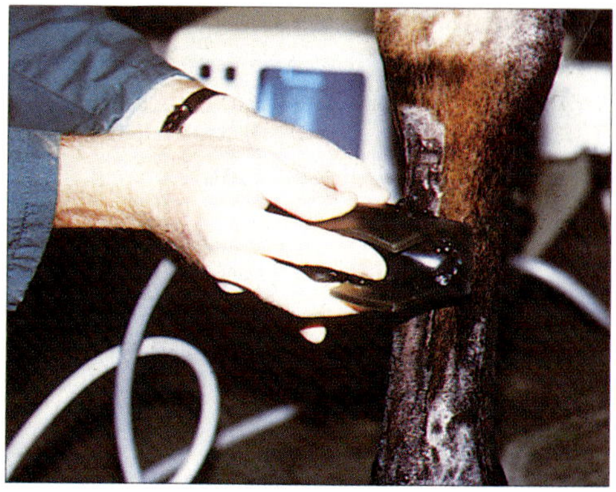

Fig. 165 *Scanning an injured tendon*

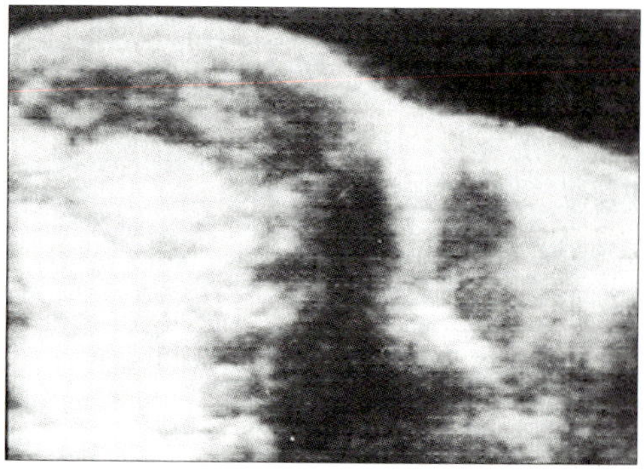

Fig. 166 *An ultra-sound scan of a tendon*
The top line is the skin, with the flexor tendons and suspensory ligaments lying progressively deeper down the left side of the scan.

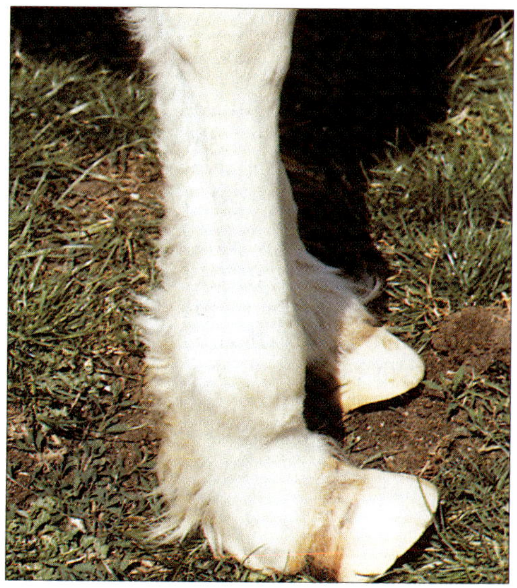

Fig. 167 *Ruptured tendon*
The fetlock lies almost flat on the floor in this case.

Stifle bone cysts

Symptoms Stifle lameness may be accompanied by swelling of the joint capsule. On X-ray cystic cavities are seen in the bone at the end of the femur.

Cause Unknown.

Treatment Many horses become sound with prolonged rest. Surgery may be attempted by opening up the cyst and filling it with a bone graft.

Prognosis Fair.

Stifle osteochondritis

Symptoms A sudden painless swelling of the capsule around the stifle joint. The horse is lame, and this is increased by flexing the leg. On X-ray, a piece of bone is often seen floating in the joint. *(Fig. 168).*

Cause Unknown.

Treatment Surgical removal of any bone fragments and damaged cartilage will be necessary.

Prognosis Fair.

Stringhalt

Symptoms Excessive and sudden bending of the hock as the horse walks. It is exaggerated if the horse is made to turn or go backwards.

Cause In isolated cases it is due to degeneration of nerves. Plant toxicity can cause the condition and give rise to several cases in the same grazing area.

Treatment Symptoms may be reduced by removing a portion of the tendon of the lateral digital extensor muscle as it passes down the side of the hock, i.e. the muscle which causes the characteristic movement. If plant toxicity is suspected, the horse must be taken off the grazing.

Prognosis Fair.

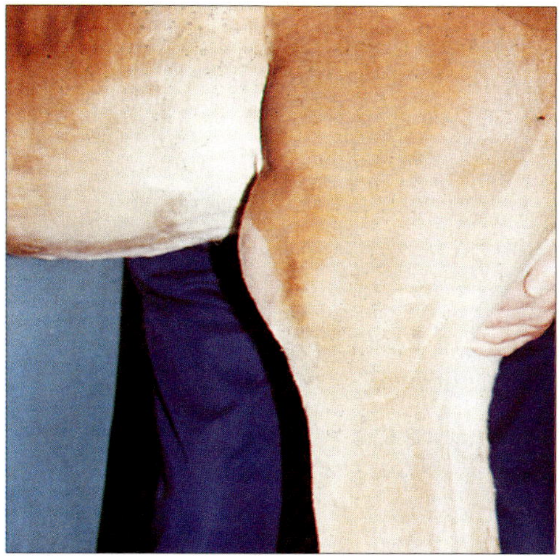

Fig. 168 *Osteochondritis of the stifle*
The joint is very swollen, but is not painful to the touch.

Suspensory ligament sprain

Symptoms Lameness associated with swelling in front of the lower third of the flexor tendons or above the sesamoid bones. An ultrasound scan may confirm the diagnosis. The ligament is thickened.

Cause A sprain of the suspensory ligament or its medial and lateral branches.

Treatment As for tendon sprain.

Prognosis Poor, especially for a return to jumping.

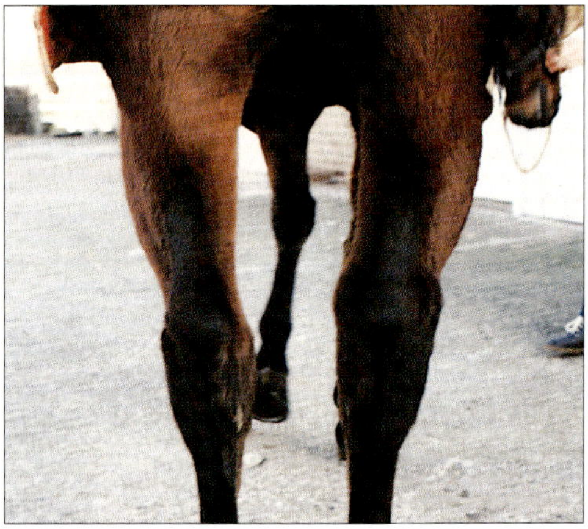

Fig. 169 *Thoroughpin*
Note the swelling just above the point of the hock of the affected leg.

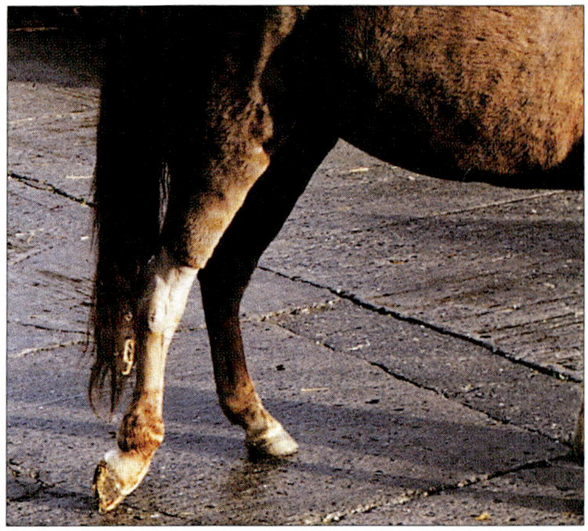

Fig. 170 *A horse with a locked patella*

Thoroughpin

Symptoms A painless swelling of the sheath of the deep flexor tendon as it passes upwards and forwards from the hock, i.e. underneath the Achilles tendon *(Fig. 169).* The horse is not lame.

Cause Possibly due to slightly increased strain as a result of poor conformation.

Treatment No treatment is usually necessary, although draining of the fluid and replacement with corticosteroids has been successful in removing the blemish.

Prognosis Good.

Thrush

Symptoms The foot has a foul smell. The horn of the frog and/or the grooves around it are soft and black. The foot may be warm and the horse lame.

Cause An infection of the horn with bacteria, helped by softening of the horn due to damp stable conditions.

Treatment Removal of infected horn is followed by daily applications of formalin solution to kill the infection and harden the horn. Stable hygiene must be improved.

Prognosis Good.

Upward fixation of the patella

Symptoms The hind leg locks while straight out behind the horse *(Fig. 170).* It may remain locked for hours or it may happen only intermittently. Walking uphill exacerbates the problem, as does trotting off suddenly from standstill.

Cause There may be a hereditary predisposition to the problem. The patella is locked in the position used to hold the leg rigid while the horse is standing or sleeping, i.e. with the medial ligament from the patella 'hooked over' the medial trochlea at the end of the femur. In horses in poor condition, the ligaments may shorten so that it is harder for the horse to avoid the patella locking at every stride.

Treatment If a nutritional involvement is suspected, food intake must be improved. If fixation is a recurring problem, surgery is necessary. This involves cutting the medial patellar ligament.

Prognosis Good.

Valgus/varus

Symptoms A lateral (valgus) or medial (varus) deviation of the lower foreleg *(Fig. 171)*. It appears in foals during the first year of life. The condition is not painful.

Cause Uneven growth of one or more growth plates in the immature bone.

Treatment In the very early stages, corrective foot trimming may bring the leg back into the vertical. Many cases require surgery either to restrict or stimulate one side of the growth plate.

Prognosis Once the growth plates disappear with maturity, the condition is permanent.

Windgalls

Symptoms A soft, cold swelling extending upwards from the back of the fetlock, between the tendons and the cannon bone *(Fig. 172)*. Lameness is rare. Often, two or more legs are affected.

Cause A stretching of the joint capsule of the fetlock and an increase in the amount of joint fluid it contains is a response to repeated mild inflammation. Faulty conformation may sometimes be a factor.

Treatment Pressure bandaging may give a temporary 'cure', but the windgall will usually recur.

Prognosis Good, in the sense that the condition does not affect the horse's usefulness.

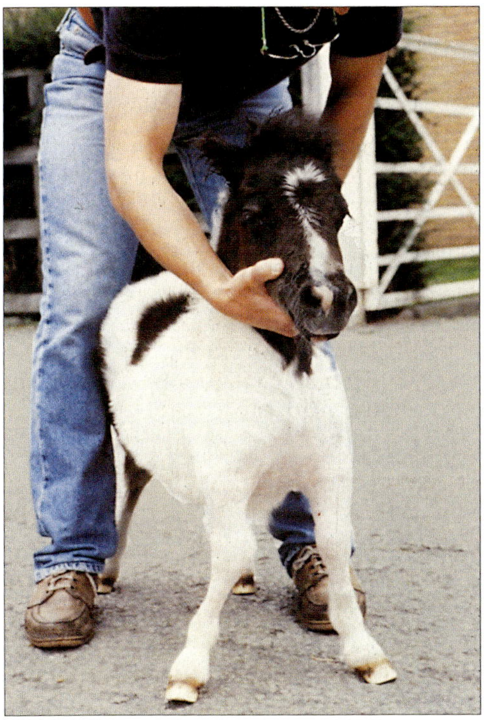

Fig. 171 A valgus deformity in the foal's forelegs.

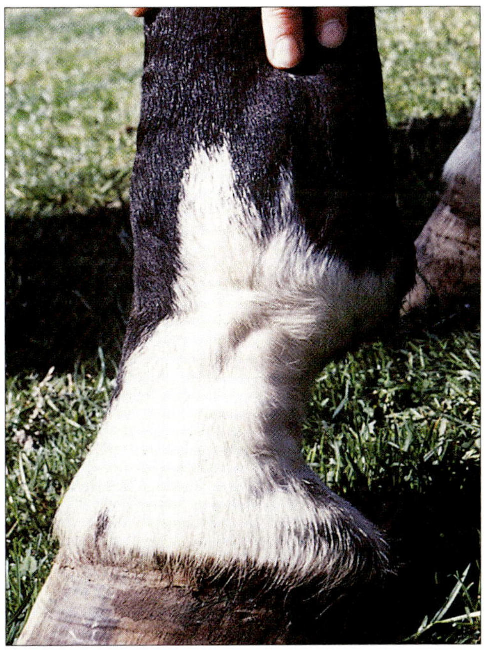

Fig. 172 *Windgalls*
The swelling extends up the back of the leg from the fetlock joint.

Veterinary Governing Bodies

Australia
Australian Capital Territory: The Registrar, Veterinary Surgeons Board of the Australian Capital Territory, PO Box 1309, Tuggeranong, ACT 2900.

New South Wales: The Registrar, Veterinary Surgeons Board of NSW, Locked Bag 21, Orange, NSW 2800.

Northern Territory: The Registrar, Veterinary Surgeons Board of the Northern Territory, c/o Department of Primary Industry and Fisheries, GPO Box 990, Darwin, Northern Territory 0801.

Queensland: The Registrar, Veterinary Surgeons Board of Queensland, Primary Industries Building, 80 Ann Street, Brisbane, Queensland 4000. (Correspondence GPO Box 46, Brisbane, Queensland 4001.)

South Australia: The Registrar, South Australian Veterinary Surgeons Board, Suite 13, 70 Walkerville Terrace, Walkerville, South Australia 5081, (PO Box 201, North Adelaide, South Australia 5006.)

Tasmania: The Registrar, Veterinary Board of Tasmania, Department of Primary Industry and Fisheries, PO Box 180, Kings Meadows, Tasmania 7249.

Victoria: The Registrar, Veterinary Board of Victoria, 272 Brunswick Road, Brunswick, Victoria 3056.

Western Australia: The Registrar, Veterinary Surgeons Board, 28 Charles Street, South Perth, Western Australia 6151.

Canada
Executive Director, Canadian Veterinary Medical Association, 339 Booth Street, Ottawa KIR 7KI, Ontario.

Republic of Ireland
Patrick J. O'Connor, MVB, MRCVS, Registrar, Veterinary Council, 53 Lansdowne Road, Ballsbridge, Dublin 4.

New Zealand
The Secretary, Veterinary Surgeons Board of New Zealand, 95B Bank House, 101-103 The Terrace, PO Box 10563, Wellington.

South Africa
The Registrar, South African Veterinary Council, PO Box 873, Pretoria 0001.

United Kingdom
Royal College of Veterinary Surgeons, Belgravia House, 62 Horseferry Road, London W1P 2AF.

United States
American Veterinary Medical Association (AVMA), 1931 North Meacham Road, Suite 100, Schaumburg, IL 60173-4360.

American Association of Equine Practitioners (AAEP), 4075 Iron Works Pike, Lexington, KY 40511.

American Horse Council, 1700 K Street NW, Suite 300, Washington, DC 20006.

Index

A

B

C

D